PIZZA

Acknowledgements

I would like to thank my friends and family for their support. And of course you for reading my book. I truly do appreciate it. Thank you so much.

Happy reading,

Adam Bryan
Author

Introduction

Hey, what's up? I'm Adam Bryan, the author of this book, and if you ever asked yourself:

> *"What restaurants offer gluten free options?"*

> *"Are there any restaurants that almost eliminate the risk of cross-contamination?"*

> *"What on earth can I eat at McDonalds, Taco Bell, or any other fast food restaurant?"*

> *"Since I'm a Celiac, can I eat out safely?"*

> *"How can I eat at a restaurant comfortably without getting sick?"*

> *"Where can I get a juicy cheeseburger on a freshly baked bun?"*

> *Or if you've ever just needed to just get awesome, trustworthy gluten free dining information...*

...I can assure you that you're in the **RIGHT** book!

Eating out can be hard...I wrote this restaurant guide to make it a heck of a lot easier.

Gluten free dining is so difficult. Trust me, I've been there.

I've been to those restaurants when your waiter/waitress brings you a basket of warm, fresh bread with salted butter even after you clearly told your them that you absolutely can't have gluten or bread of any sort.

I've been to that restaurant where your server brings you a juicy hamburger on fresh bun instead of that lettuce wrap you clearly requested.

And I've definitely been to that restaurant where the chef and manager comes out stating that they'll be sure to accommodate your gluten free diet, when you clearly see that clueless look on their face as they try to remember what you can and can't eat.

It's hard and sometimes it just plain sucks.

But that will now change. Why?

You have this gluten free Bible of sorts.

You now have the key to a stress-free gluten dining experience in the palm of your hands.

You see, I decided to give you gluten free foodies a hand by listing **complete** gluten free menus from almost all major eating chained establishments from across the nation.

Red Lobster? Check.

McDonalds? Check

Starbucks? Check.

And hundreds more just a few pages away.

In this book, you'll discover gluten free menus from most major fast food and table-service restaurants across the United States.

Plus, I'll also teach you some killer dining tips that I know will help make eating out gluten-free a whole lot easier for you.

You see, I'm just your gluten free restaurant middleman.

I've researched and discovered all the gluten free chain restaurant menus available and I brought them all to one, easy to navigate, straightforward book- created just for you.

If you're ready to stop worrying about cross-contamination or any of those other hassles of ordering gluten free options from restaurants, but instead start enjoying the relaxed restaurant life where you're constantly stuffing your face, turn the page.

Happiness awaits... and by happiness, I mean a full belly.

What is Gluten?

Okay, let me go all scientific on you guys for a second.

The term "gluten" technically refers to a specific complex of proteins that forms when wheat flour is mixed with a liquid and physically manipulated, such as in the kneading of bread. The Food and Drug Administration (FDA) is proposing to define the term "gluten" to mean the proteins that naturally occur in a prohibited grain (see below) and that may cause adverse health effects in persons with celiac disease.

In a more simplified definition, gluten is what most scientists like to call a storage protein. Its what gives dough the elastic texture and feel to it.

Prolamins are a class of proteins present in a variety of grains, and they're what cause problems for people who can't eat gluten.

Gluten has become a more general term for any kind of potentially harmful prolamin.

The prolamins that tend to cause damage to people with celiac disease or any other gluten allergies include gliadin, found in wheat, secalin, found in rye, and horedin, found in barley.

Here's a definition so easy a 1st grader would understand it.

Gluten is what makes bread stretchy and "elastic-y."

Popular Foods & Drinks that Have Gluten in Them

Gluten is not just found in bread and other things that contain wheat or barley. Gluten can be found in places you'd least expect.

Here are the most popular foods that have gluten in them that you'll find in most restaurants. The list includes typical food/drink items, not special gluten-free version, just to be clear.

1. Bread

Most sandwich breads, Paninis, wraps, submarine rolls, dinner rolls, and hamburger/hot dog buns contain gluten.

2. Beer

Most beer contains gluten, unless you are drinking a specialty brew like grapefruit beer or butter beer. But other than that, always be sure to avoid beer unless you opt for a gluten free beer, such as Red Bridge or Bards, just to name a few.

3. Salad (Croutons & Some Dressings)

Okay let me be clear. Plain salads with just raw vegetables are gluten free. The tricky part happens when you start adding croutons and the dressing. As most croutons contain gluten, you should be sure to order your salad minus croutons. Now in terms of dressing, some of them have gluten in them. Just be sure to do your research. A word of advice, watch out for cream based dressings, more specially bleu cheese. It's a risky one.

4. Chips

Most chips contain gluten unless it's corn tortilla chips. So if you're ever at a Mexican restaurant that offers chips and salsa, there's a good chance that those chips are safe. But always ask your server

5. Baked Goods

Pastries, cakes, cookies, brownies, and cannoli's all contain gluten in them. However, if you're ever at a restaurant that offers a flourless cake or brownie such as Bonefish Grill, you're in the clear so dig in!

6. Crackers

Whenever you order soup at a restaurant, be sure to not add crackers to it because they contain gluten

7. Licorice

Twizzlers, Red Vines, and other licorice treats contain wheat aka gluten. Gummy bears and most gummy candies are safe though! Always check the ingredient lists however just to be safe.

8. Pasta

Most wheat-based pastas contain gluten. The only time they don't is if you order rice noodles. Thankfully many Italian restaurants offer gluten-free pasta!

9. Pizza

Pizza from the big/popular pizza joints including Pizza Hut and Papa Johns contain gluten. The same goes for some smaller ones. Thankfully some smaller pizza chains offer gluten free pizza. Plus, Dominos has one too! (Not safe for the gluten allergenic, however.)

10. Pretzels

Don't get suckered in to a crab-stuffed soft pretzel or pretzel bites. Pretzels contain gluten.

11. Hamburger Meat

Some restaurants like to add bread crumbs to their hamburgers so be sure to ask you server if there is gluten in the hamburger meat before you order.

12. Meatballs

Don't let the name fool you. Meatballs contain breadcrumbs and wheat. So always stay clear or at least ask your server first.

13. Soy Sauce

Is your mind blown yet? Yes, soy sauce contains gluten so be sure to watch out when you go out to eat at any Asian restaurant because chances are, there's soy sauce in your meal, especially in fried rice.

7 Gluten Free Dining Tips from the Pros

I'm a terrible cook.

Like seriously, I don't know how to cook a single thing. Wait, actually I do know how to make scrambled eggs, but that's it. It's sad, I know.

But what I do know is how to eat. I like to call myself a full-time eater because 8 hours of my day is usually spent eating, and the other 8 hours is usually spent thinking about what to eat. (The other 8 hours is usually spent taking my online college course, *"Sleepology 101"* where I study the back of my eyelids. You should all definitely take it next semester!)

Since I don't cook, I usually eat out at restaurants or fast food joints for almost all my meals. Luckily for me, I live and breathe gluten free restaurant menus so trying to determine what I can eat at a particular restaurant comes naturally to me.

But there's a lot more to just finding a gluten free menu item and ordering. There are a lot more steps and things you should do in order to create the best gluten free dining experience for yourself.

There are quite a few things you should consider doing while eating out at restaurants. But you don't want to hear these gluten free dining tips just from just me right?

What better way to discover new ways to dine out gluten free than hear it from the pros themselves!

Below, I gathered 7, extremely simple yet effective gluten free dining tips from some of the most prolific, successful, influential gluten free bloggers, authors, and bakers around. And thankfully they were all willing to share a tip or two to help make your gluten free dining out experience a little bit better. Enjoy!

1. Always eat before you head out to the restaurant.

Amie Valpone, from The Healthy Apple

"My Tip for Eating Out: Always eat before you head out to the restaurant so that you're not eyeing the bread basket while everyone else is diving in. I tell my clients to bring their own gluten-free crackers such as Crunchmaster Crackers to restaurants to enjoy before their meal if they miss bread baskets. Eating before you head to the restaurant won't leave you ravenous and if the restaurant of your choice is booked and you have to go somewhere else that doesn't have any gluten-free items- you won't be starving and you'll be able to enjoy yourself until you can find food when you leave the restaurant!"

2. Eat at gluten friendly restaurants

Karina, from Gluten Free Goddess

"In my opinion, there are 2 types of gluten friendly restaurants: restaurants with a gluten free menu; and restaurants with a designated gluten free kitchen. You can check out all the restaurants with a gluten free menu here, plus you can also find some gluten free kitchens in your state by checking out this page on Celiac Central. Bon appetit!

3. Talk to the waiter about the safest choice on the menu

Karina, from Gluten Free Goddess

"I rarely eat out- but if I do I only eat at a gluten-free friendly restaurant; I talk to the waiter as an ally advising what would be the safest choice on the menu (a good waiter will know- a bad waiter won't care; if I don't feel comfortable, I don't order anything)."

4. Talk to the managers/chefs and ask for an ingredients list.

Jules, from Jules Gluten Free and the Jules Speaks Gluten Free Blog

"...Always talk to managers or chefs is a start! Also check for full ingredient list & how cross-contamination [is] prevented."

5. Tell the waiter

Cathy, from Strawberries are Gluten Free

"Tell the waiter! And because gfree is now somewhat popular it is more important than ever to differentiate. I encourage you to word it like this: "I have a severe allergy to gluten... Similar to a peanut allergy. Would you let the cook know please?" yes, its not technically correct but it gets an easy to understand nessage across to a layperson.

Sometimes humor works too, 'If i so much as smell gluten Ill be tying up your bathroom for the entire afternoon'."

6. Try eating at fast food or higher end restaurants

Cathy, from Strawberries Are Gluten Free

"You'll have a safer experience at high end or fast food restaurants for very different reasons. Fast food restaurants because of the assembly line procedures where cross contamination isunlikely even if none of them have any idea what celiacs is. And high end restaurants because theyre generally more educated and accommodating of special requests."

7. Call ahead.

Jamie, from Gluten Free Mom

"Unless you have eaten at the restaurant before, call ahead and make sure they can accommodate your diet and find out exactly what they can make for you. Do not rely on the hostess – ask to speak directly to the Chef. If not available, then ask for the kitchen manager. Insist on knowing what they can prepare safely – don't stop at a "rest assured we can cook for you."

My thoughts...

Wow, these tips were killer! I agree with every single one of them. So, with that being said, I hope you enjoyed these 7 helpful gluten free dining tips from the pros themselves.

Warning! Read Before You Eat!

Although these restaurants provide gluten free menu items and menus, they do encourage anyone with food sensitivities, allergies, or special dietary needs to consult with a medical professional for informed answers relating to their specific sensitivities and the risks involved when dining out.

Also please be aware that some food will be in the presence of gluten items, such as in burger joints and delis, so please be advised and use caution.

Also, please be sure to alert the restaurant that you have a gluten allergy so that they can take the proper measures to avoid any cross contamination.

Please understand that most, if not all restaurants cannot be completely free of allergens. So please be careful.

ALSO BE SURE TO NOTIFY YOUR SERVER AND THE RESTAURANT THAT YOU HAVE A GLUTEN ALLERGY, SENSITIVITY, OR DIETARY NEED.

Your body will seriously thank you.

The Gluten Free Restaurant Menus

In terms of restaurant menu updates, these menus are only valid as of 1/3/2014. You will find new, up to date versions of these gluten free menus in the future on my website, ***www.GlutenFreeGuideHQ.com***. So be sure to always check the site for any new menus, including new updates.

Thankfully, many of these gluten free options tend to stay the same for the rest of the year.

Menu Accuracy

100% of all the menus and menu items were gathered directly from the restaurant chains themselves. This means that everything you see on the gluten free menus in this book came directly from the corporate offices of these chain restaurants.

There is no guessing or assumptions on my part. Your health and safety is my biggest concern so I want to make sure that I provide you with the most accurate gluten free listing possible.

I even made sure to add some safety and ordering tips to help make your gluten free dining experience safer.

Alright, so let's get started!

Burgers & Fries

Burgers and fries anyone? I know what you're thinking. You're probably thinking that all these burger joints only wrap your burger in lettuce or worst, just throw it on a plate and serve it to you. But let me tell you, you'd be quite surprised about the delicious burgers WITH a gluten free bun that you can find across the U.S. It's now time to enjoy burgers the way they were meant to be enjoyed – with a warm fresh gluten free bun!

Arby's

Meats

- Black Angus Roast Beef
- Corned Beef
- Genoa Salami
- Pecan Chicken Salad+
- Pepper Bacon
- Pepperoni
- Roast Beef
- Roast Chicken+
- Roast Ham Roast Turkey

Sides

- Applesauce

Salads

- Chopped Farmhouse Salad-Turkey & Ham
- Chopped Farmhouse Chicken-Roast
- Chopped Side Salad

Condiments

- Arby's Sauce®
- Banana Peppers
- Chargrill Seasoning
- Cheddar Cheese Sauce+
- Cheddar Cheese, Sharp Natural Slice
- Cheddar Cheese, Shredded Natural
- Cheddar Cheese, Processed Slice
- Dijon Honey Mustard Sandwich Sauce
- Dill Pickle Slices
- Horsey Sauce®
- Ketchup
- Mayonnaise
- Parmesan Peppercorn Ranch Sauce
- Pecan Chicken Salad
- Pepper & Onion Mix
- Red Ranch Sauce
- Red Wine Vinaigrette Sauce
- Sauerkraut
- Smoky Q Sauce*
- Spicy Brown Honey Mustard Sauce
- Swiss Cheese, Big Eye Natural
- Swiss Cheese, Processed Slice
- Thousand Island Spread
- Yellow Mustard

Dressings

- Balsamic Vinaigrette Dressing
- Buttermilk Ranch Dressing
- Dijon Honey Mustard Dressing
- Light Italian Dressing

Dipping Sauces

- Buffalo Sauce

- Honey Dijon Mustard Sauce
- Ranch Sauce
- Tangy Barbeque Sauce
- Bronco Berry Sauce®

Beverages

- 1% Low Fat Chocolate Milk
- 2% Reduced Fat Milk
- CapriSun® Fruit Juice
- Coffee
- Diet Pepsi®
- Dr Pepper®
- Mountain Dew®
- Pepsi®
- Sierra Mist®
- Brewed Iced Tea
- Nestlé® Pure Life® Bottled Water

Desserts

- Chocolate Shake
- Jamocha Swirl Shake
- Vanilla Shake

Backyard Burger

Burgers

Be sure to order all burgers without a bun.

- Back Yard American Cheeseburger
- Back Yard Bleu Cheeseburger
- Back Yard Cheddar Cheeseburger
- Backyard Pepper Jack Cheeseburger

- Backyard Swiss CheeseBurger
- Bacon Cheddar Burger
- Mushroom Swiss Burger
- Garden Veggie Burger

Chicken Sandwiches

Be sure to order all chicken sandwiches without a bun.

- Blackened Chicken
- Grilled Chicken

Specialty Items

- Back Yard Hot Dog without Bun
- Bak Pak Dog without Bun
- Chili Cheese Big Dog without Bun

Salads

Be sure to order all salads without croutons

- Blackened Chicken Salad
- Garden Fresh Salad
- Grilled Chicken Salad

Sides

- Chili
- Side Salad

Dressings and Sauces

- Honey Mustard
- Bleu Cheese
- Ranch
- Lite Ranch
- Margarine Cup

- Lite Mayonnaise
- Mayonnaise

Desserts and Shakes

- Ice Cream a la mode
- Chocolate Shake
- Strawberry Shake
- Vanilla Shake

Bareburgers

Meats

- Beef
- Turkey
- Farmers Quinoa Veggie Burger
- Mushroom Burger
- Blackbean Burger
- Buttermilk Fried Chicken
- Grilled or Jerk Chicken
- Lamb
- Wild Boar
- Elk
- Bison
- Ostrich

Bread

- Tapioca Rice Bun

Veggies

- Iceberg lettuce
- Red raw onions

- Tomatoes
- Garlic dill pickle chips
- Fire roasted red peppers
- Sweet apple
- Grilled Onions
- Sauteed Mushrooms
- Fried Egg
- Has
- Avocado

Cheese

- Colby
- Sharp Cheddar
- Pepperjack
- Smoked Mozzarella
- Wisconsin Blue
- Vegan Cheddar

Bacon

- Applewood Smoked Thick Cut Bacon
- County Bacon
- Turkey Bacon
- Hardwood Smoked Brisket

Sauce

- Ketchup
- Mayo
- Stone Ground Mustard
- Curry ketchup
- Bareburger Special Sauce Habanero
- Chipotle Mayo
- Smokehouse Sauce
- Smoked Paprika Mayo
- Buttermilk Rnach

- Stone Ground Honey Mustard
- Salsa Verde
- Buffalo Sauce
- Basil Pesto
- Bacon Marmalade

Bare Snacks

- Assorted Pickles

Bare Salads

- Farmers
- Mexican
- Cranberry Blue
- Asian
- Poached Pear
- Italian
- Cobb
- Walnut Apple

Bare Sides

- Small house salad
- House-made Carolina slaw
- Spicy pickle chips
- Garlic dill pickle chips
- Butter pickle chips

Bare Sweets

- Flourless Chocolate Cake
- Kids Sundae
- Banana Foster Milkshake
- Root Beer Float
- Hot Honey Milkshake

Bare Shakes

- Vanilla
- Chocolate
- Peanut Butter
- Banana
- Strawberry
- Raspberry

Burger 21

Certified Angus Beef Burgers

All of Burger 21's gluten-free burgers are served on a French Meadow Bakery Gluten-Free bun.

- Burger 101
- Cheesy Burger
- Bacon Cheesy Burger
- The Shroom
- Black and Bleu
- Philly Cheese
- The OMG!

Fries

- French Fries
- Sweet Potato Fries
- Half and Half (a combo of both regular and sweet potato fries)

Fresh Salads

- The Chopped Cobb
- Black and Bleu Wedge
- The Sonoma Valley
- Super Burger Bowl

- Side Garden Salad

Salad Dressings

- raspberry walnut vinaigrette
- red wine vinaigrette
- ranch
- honey mustard
- avocado ranch

Kid's Menu

- Burger Cheesy Burger
- Garden Salad
- Kiddie Sundae

Hand Dipped Shakes

- Vanilla Bean
- Chocolate
- Strawberry
- Bananas Foster
- Ybor City Double Espresso
- Chocolate Peanut Butter

Retro Floats

- Coke
- Boylan Birch Beer,
- Boylan Créme
- Boylan Black Cherry,
- Boylan Root Beer
- Boylan Orange

Burgerville

Salads

- Wild Smoked Salmon and Hazelnut Salad
- Grilled Chicken Salad
- Side Salad

Sides

Be sure to ask if any other foods are cooked in the same fryers as the french fries and hash browns.

- French Fries
- Hash-browns
- Sliced Apples

Dipping Sauces and Salad Dressings

- BBQ Sauce
- Honey Mustard
- Blue Cheese Dressing
- Raspberry Vinaigrette
- Ranch Dressing
- Balsamic Vinaigrette
- Tartar Sauce

Desserts

- All milkshakes and smoothies
- Sundaes

Checkers

Classic Wings

- Honey BBQ
- Medium Buffalo

Milkshakes

- Vanilla
- Chocolate
- Strawberry
- Banana

Cheeseburger in Paradise

For all sandwiches, be sure to order a gluten free bun!

First Wave aka Appetizers

- Black Angus Sliders: Order without buns
- Loaded Chips

Sunset Salads and Soups

- Calypso Chicken Salad: Order with grilled Chicken
- Son of a Sailor Salad
- Costa Rican Steak Salad: Order without wontons.

Paradise Specialties

- BBQ Ribs
- St. Barts Citrus Chicken: Order without Island Rice or Teriyaki Broccoli

- Parrot Beach Salmon: Order without Island Rice or Teriyaki Broccoli

Cheeseburgers in Paradise

"We are proud to serve our New Gluten Free Bun for any of our burgers for $1.00 extra. A turkey and Veggie Burger can be substituted at no additional cost (Both are gluten free)."

- Bacon Cheddar Burger
- Baja Burger
- Mini-Cheeseburgers: Order without buns
- BBQ Bacon Burger
- All-American Beach Burger
- Black Angus Beef Burger

Surfside Sandwiches

- BBQ Chicken Sandwich: Order gluten free bun
- Fish Sandwich: Order gluten free bun

Sides

- French fried potatoes
- Vegetable of the day
- Coleslaw

Little Parakeets aka Kids Menu

Includes a choice of a beverage (soda, milk, or fresh parakeet punch) and a choice of a side (French fried potatoes, coleslaw, or mandarin oranges).

- Mini-Cheeseburgers: order without buns
- Grilled Chicken Breast
- BBQ Ribs
- Grilled Flame Steak

Sensuous Treats

- Copa Banana: Order without Nilla Wafers
- Lil' Pirates Treat: Order without Oreo cookie crumbles

Tiki Bar Favorites

- C.I.P Cocktail
- Blackberry Sangria
- House Piña Colada
- Pink Flamingo Rita
- Tropical Island Tea
- Red Bridge

Non-Alcoholic Beverages

- Hand-Dipped Milkshakes
- Island Paradise
- Jamaican Root Beer Float
- Surfside Sodas
- Flavored Iced Tea: Peach, Mango, Pomegranate, Raspberry and Blueberry
- Sodas (Coke, Diet Coke, Sprite, Fresca, Coke Zero, Barq's Root Beer)

Other Drinks

- Strawberry Lemonade
- Island Lemonade
- Lemonade Iced Tea
- Brewed Iced Tea
- Freshly Brewed Coffee
- Bottled Water
- Red Bull

Dairy Queen

When you are getting a Blizzard, please understand that the mixer is used for all flavors so there is a chance of cross contamination. So as a result, Dairy Queen urges you to request that the crew clean the mixer prior to making your blizzard.

Treats

- Chocolate or Vanilla soft served in a cup
- DQ Fudge Bar
- DQVanilla
- Orange Bar
- Dilly Bars (all flavors)
- Buster Bar Treat
- Starkiss Bars (all flavors) – in a sealed plastic wrapper
- Sundaes: Chocolate, Caramel, Hot Fudge, Marshmallow, and Strawberry

Blizzard Treats

- Reese's Peanut Butter Cup
- Butterfinger
- Heath
- M&M's
- Banana Split
- Hawaiian
- Tropical

Drinks

- Arctic Rush slush (all flavors)
- MooLatté frozen blended coffee drinks (vanilla, caramel, mocha)
- Shakes: Chocolate, Caramel, Hot Fudge, Marshmallow, and Strawberry
- All flavors of fountain soda

Food

- French Fries (fried with foods containing gluten so cross-contamination exists)
- Grilled Chicken patty ordered without bun
- Hamburger patty ordered without bun
- GrillBurger patty ordered without bun
- Hot Dog frank ordered without bun

Fatburger

Burgers and Sandwiches

Be sure to order with no buns.

- Fatburger with no bun

Salads

- Fat Salad Wedge with no dressing
- Fat Salad Wedge with Chicken and no dressing

Fries

- Big Fat Fries
- Chili Cheese Skinny Fries
- Chilly Cheese Fat Fries
- Chili Skinny Fries
- Chili Fat Fries

Sides

- Chili Cup
- Chili Cup with Cheese and Onions

Add Ons

- Cheddar Cheese
- Egg
- Bacon
- Chili
- American Cheese

Toppings

- Mayonnaise
- Lettuce
- Tomato
- Pickles
- Onions
- Grilled Onions
- Relish
- Mustard

Shakes

- Vanilla
- Chocolate
- Strawberry
- Maui-Banana
- Big Fat Float

Five Guys

All burgers and hot dogs must be ordered without the bun. My suggestion is to go ahead and bring your own gluten-free bun from home.

Burgers

- Hamburger
- Cheeseburger
- Bacon Burger
- Bacon Cheeseburger
- Little Hamburger
- Little Cheeseburger

- Little Bacon Burger
- Little Bacon Cheeseburger

Dogs (Hot Dogs)

Order without buns

- Kosher Style Hot Dog
- Cheese Dog
- Bacon Dog
- Bacon Cheese Dog

Sandwiches

Order without buns. Veggie Sandwiches do not contain veggie burger patties.

- Veggie Sandwich
- Cheese Veggie Sandwich

Fries

- Five Guys Style
- Cajun Style

100% Free Toppings

- Mayo
- Lettuce
- Pickles
- Tomatoes
- Grilled Onions
- Grilled Mushrooms
- Ketchup
- Mustard
- Relish
- Onions
- Jalapeno Peppers
- Green Peppers
- A1 Steak Sauce
- Bar-B-Q Sauce
- Hot Sauce

Freddys

Burgers and Dogs

Be sure to order these items "protein style" wrapped in lettuce or on a bed of lettuce for a salad. Plus the Freddys Signature Seasoning is gluten free so you don't have to worry about that.

- Steakburgers
- Hot Dogs

Fries

Cross contamination exists since these fries are fried in the smae fryer as chicken strips and onion rings. Celiacs or anyone with an allergy should not eat the fries.

- French Fries

Chili

The chili contains oats and modified food starch however, it is still gluten free. Not celiac and gluten allergen friendly.

- Chili

Special Sauces

- Gehl's Cheese Sauce

Dessert and Toppings

- Custard
- Hot Fudge
- Caramel
- Butterscotch
- Marshmallow

- Peanut Butter
- Banana
- Cherry
- Pineapple
- Butterfinger
- M&Ms

In N Out Burger

Burgers

Be sure to order all burgers protein style (aka wrapped in lettuce) or animal style (wrapped in lettuce but with pickles, tomatoes, onions, etc.) as seen on their secret menu.

- Hamburger
- Cheeseburger

Fries

The only fried in the fryers are french fries so cross contamination is virtually non-existent. Hooray!

- French Fries

Shakes

- Vanilla
- Chocolate
- Strawberry

Jack In the Box

Entrees

- Grilled chicken strips (4 pc)

Salads

- Chicken Club Salad w/Grilled Chicken Strips
- Grilled Chicken Salad
- Side Salad
- Southwest Chicken Salad w/Grilled Chicken Strips

Salad Dressings

- Creamy Southwest Dressing
- Lite Ranch Dressing
- Low Fat Balsamic Vinagrette Dressing
- Spicy Corn Sticks
- Hearty Breakfast Bowl

Sides

- Hashbrown Sticks (5 pc.)
- Chiquita® Apple Bites with caramel

Sauces and Condiments

- Buttermilk House Dipping Sauce
- Fire Roasted Salsa
- Frank's
- RedHot
- Buffalo Dipping Sauce
- Honey Mustard Dipping Sauce
- Log Cabin®
- Syrup

- Sweet & Sour Dipping Sauce
- Tartar Sauce
- Zesty Marinara Sauce
- Substitute Sauces Allergens Soy Egg Fish Milk Peanuts
- Chipotle Sauce
- Creamy Italian Sauce
- Creamy Ranch Sauce
- Ketchup
- Mayo-Onion
- Mustard
- Peppercorn Mayo
- Sun Dried Tomato Sauce
- Fire Roasted Salsa
- Grape Jelly
- Grilled Onions
- Ketchup
- Malt Vinegar
- Mayonnaise
- Mustard
- Pride Margarine Spread
- Red Onion
- Secret Sauce
- Sour Cream
- Strawberry Jelly
- Taco Sauce
- Drinks and Beverages
- All drinks and beverages

Desserts

- Blackberry Shake with Whipped Topping
- Strawberry Shake with Whipped Topping
- Vanilla Shake with Whipped Topping

Krystal Burger

Burgers

Be sure to order without the bun. And watch out for cross contamination.

- Angus Burger Patty
- Krystal Beef Patty

Meats

- Pup Frank
- Bacon
- Sausage
- Sunrise Sausage
- Whole Eggs

Sides

- French Fries
- Potato Kryspers
- Grits
- Quick Grits

Toppings and Add Ons

- Cheese Slice
- Chopped Onions
- Dill Chips
- Lettuce Blend
- Mayonnaise
- Mustard
- Ketchup
- Jalapenos
- Sauces
- Sweet & Spicy BBQ Sauce

- Ranch
- Honey
- Kens Steak House Cannonball BBQ Sauce
- Kens Steak House Country French with Vermont Honey
- Honey Dijon Dressing
- Lite Italian Dressing
- Spicy Wing
- Sweet & Spicy Honey Mustard

Milkshakes

- Chocolate
- Strawberry
- Vanilla

McDonalds

Meats

- Beef Patty with no bun
- Breakfast Beef Steak
- Canadian Bacon
- Sausage
- Scrambled Egg

Side

- Fruit 'n Yogurt Parfait with no granola

McDonald's Salads

- McDonalds Premium Bacon Ranch Salad with grilled Chicken (gluten-free)
- Caesar Salad w/o Chicken
- Premium Bacon Ranch Salad

- Premium Southwest Salad (without tortilla strips)
- Side Salad

McDonald's Dressings

- Newman's Own Creamy Caesar Dressing
- Newman's Own Cobb Dressing
- Newman's Own Low Fat Balsamic Vinaigrette
- Newman's Own Ranch Dressing
- Newman's Own Salsa

Drinks, Beverages, and Desserts

- Apple Juice
- Coffee
- Hot Chocolate
- 1% Low Fat Milk, White or Chocolate
- Orange Juice
- Soft Drinks

Desserts

- Chocolate Triple Thick Shake
- Strawberry Triple Thick Shake
- Vanilla Triple Thick Shake
- Ice Cream Sundaes including nuts
- McFlurry with M&M'S Candies

Sauces and Condiments

- Chicken McNugget Honey
- Chicken McNugget Hot Mustard Sauce
- Hotcake Syrup
- Jam
- Lettuce
- Mayonnaise
- Onions

- Pickles
- Tartar Sauce
- Tomato
- Apple Dippers and Low Fat Caramel Dip
- American Cheese

Milo's Hamburgers

Burgers

Without the bun

- Hamburger
- Cheeseburger
- Double Hamburger
- Double Cheeseburger

Sauces

- Milo's Sauce
- Honey Mustard

New York Fries

All fries are cooked in 100% pure sunflower oil. Plus the fries don't contain any coating. The only things that will contain any trace of gluten are the toppings and seasonings you will find on their front counter.

- Classic French Fries

Red Robin

Appetizers

- Garden Fresh Humus Plate with no garlic bread

Salads

- Simply Grilled Chicken Salad with no croutons and garlic bread
- Crispy Chicken Tender Salad with no crispy chicken (grilled chicken must be substituted) and no garlic bread
- House Salad with no croutons
- Avo-Cobb-O with no bleu cheese crumbles and no croutons
- Side Caesar Salad with no croutons or garlic bread

Salad Dressing

- Balsamic Vinaigrette Creamy Caesar
- Bleu Cheese
- Thousand Island
- Honey-Mustard Poppyseed

Fire-Grilled Burgers

All burgers MUST be ordered protein style (wrapped in lettuces instead of the bun) or with the Red Robin gluten bun.

- Red's Tavern Double
- RR Bacon Cheeseburger
- Royal Red Robin Burger
- Keep it Simple Burger
- RR Gourmet Cheeseburger

Chicken Burgers and Other Favorites

All burgers MUST be ordered protein style (wrapped in lettuces instead of the bun) or with the Red Robin gluten bun.

- Grilled Turkey Burger Simply Grilled Chicken Burger with no chipotle aioli
- Bruschetta Chicken Burger with no tomato-bruschetta salsa.

Entrees

- Ensenada Chicken Platter with no Baja Ranch Dressing, no Ancho marinade on chicken breasts, no Salsa, no tortilla strips, and no tortilla cups

Sides

- Steamed veggies
- House Salad (no croutons)
- Mandarin oranges
- Freckled Fruit Salad
- Sweet Potato Fries
- Celery sticks
- Apples

Kids Menu

- RAD Burger with a beef or turkey patty. Order protein style or with a gluten free bun
- Chick-on-a-Stick with no teriyaki sauce and no ranch

Smashburger

Meat and Protein

- Bacon
- Eggs
- Grilled Chicken Breast

Salads

- Baja Cobb
- Harvest
- Garden Salad
- Caribbean (Regional)
- Honey Mustard (Regional)
- Mediterranean (Regional)
- Miami Heat (Regional)
- Michigan Harvest (Regional)
- Spinach and Goat Cheese (Regional)
- Add Grilled Chicken to your salad

Salad Dressing

- Spicy Chipotle Dressing
- Balsamic Vinaigrette Dressing
- Honey Mustard Dressing
- Tzatziki Sauce

Sides

All these sides are cooked in a fryer that is shared with glutenous foods. So eat at your own risk. Not recommend for anyone with allergy or Celiac.

- French Fries
- Smash Fries
- Sweet Potato Fries

- Sweet Potato Smash Fries
- Veggie Frites
- Brunswick Fries (Regional)
- Cajun Fries (Regional)
- Debris Fries (Regional)
- Gravy Poutine Fries (Regional)
- Mushroom Poutine Fries (Regional)

Cheese

- American
- Cheddar
- Bleu
- Goat
- Pepper Jack
- Swiss
- Parmesan

Sauces

- Balsamic Vinaigrette
- Spicy Chipotle
- Ranch
- Ketchup
- Mayonnaise
- Spicy Brown Mustard
- Yellow Mustard
- Relish
- A-1 Sauce
- BBQ
- Franks Red Hot
- Texas Petal

Toppings

- Fried Egg
- Garlic Mushrooms

- Grilled Onions
- Guacamole

Sonic Drive In

Grill Items

- Hamburger Patty
- Bacon
- Breakfast Sausage
- Sliced Ham
- Hot Dog (Pork and Beef) without bun
- Philly Steak
- Egg
- Grilled Onions
- Red and Green Peppers

Fried Items

Cross contamination does exist since fries and tots are cooked in the same fryers as other breaded foods that contain gluten.

- French Fries
- Tots

Sides

- Fritos Corn Chips
- Apple Slices
- Sonic Mint

Other Extras

- Light Ranch
- Thousand Island Dressing
- Baja Cheese Sauce

- Carne Asada Sauce
- Ketchup
- Mustard
- Mayonnaise
- Spicy Mustard
- Hickory BBQ Sauce
- Tartar Sauce
- Celery Salt
- Salt/Pepper Blend
- Ketchup
- Mustard
- Mayonnaise
- Relish
- Tartar Sauce
- Maple Flavored Syrup
- Barbecue Sauce
- Honey Mustard Sauce
- Ranch Dressing
- Caramel Dipping Sauce
- Grape Jelly
- Strawberry Jam
- French Fry Sauce
- Sweet and Sour Sauce
- Salsa de Sonic
- Philadelphia Cream Cheese

Sandwich Toppings

- Lettuce
- Tomato
- Onion
- Sweet Pickle Relish
- Sauerkraut
- Sport Peppers
- Sliced Dill Pickle Spears
- Sliced Jalapeños

- Green Chili Peppers

Ice Cream, Add-In Flavors and Toppings

- Vanilla Ice Cream
- Milk (1% Regular and Chocolate)
- Whipped Dessert Topping
- Butterfinger
- M&M's
- Reese's
- Snickers
- Heath
- Neutral Slush Base
- Cherry Syrup
- Low-Cal Diet Cherry Syrup
- Grape Slush Syrup
- Blue Coconut Slush Syrup
- Orange Slush Syrup
- Green Apple Slush Syrup
- Watermelon Slush Syrup
- Pomegranate Blueberry Syrup
- Maraschino Cherries
- Pineapple Topping
- Strawberry Topping
- Caramel Topping
- Coconut Creme Syrup
- Cheesecake Syrup
- Chocolate Syrup
- Fresh Banana
- Peanut Butter Topping
- Nut Topping
- Chocolate Fudge Topping
- Hot Chocolate Cocoa Mix
- Raspberry Tea Syrup
- Peach Tea Syrup
- Blackberry Tea Syrup

- Mango Tea Syrup
- Mint Tea Syrup
- Lemon Juice
- Fanta Vanilla Syrup

The Counter

Starter Sauces

- Apricot sauce
- Country buttermilk ranch
- Horseradish mayo

Starters Without Sauces

- French fries
- Cheese fries
- Chili Cheese Fries
- Parmesan French Fries
- Sweet potato fries
- 50/50 Fries/Sweet
- Side Salad
- Grilled Vegetable Plate

Signature Burgers in a Bowl

- Southwester (with or without premium toppings)
- Mediterranean (with or without sundried tomatoes)

Burgers

Be sure to order with a GLUTEN FREE BUN

- Beef Burger
- Turkey Burger

Cheeses

- Yellow American
- All other cheeses except Danish Blue Cheese

Toppings

- Baby Spinach
- Bermuda Red Onion
- Black olives
- Carrot strings
- Dill pickle chips
- Dried cranberries
- Grilled onions
- Grilled pineapples
- Hard Boiled Eggs
- Jalapenos
- Lettuce blend
- Marinated artichokes
- Organic mixed greens
- Roasted Chiles
- Roasted corn and black bean salsa
- Scallions
- Sliced Cucumbers
- Spicy pepperoncinis
- Sprouts
- Tomatoes

Premium Toppings

- Applewood smoked bacon
- Avocado
- Black Forest Ham
- Chili (Beef)
- Fried Egg
- Housemade Guacamole
- Sauteed Mushrooms

- Sun-dried tomatoes

Sauces

- Apricot Sauce
- Basil Pesto
- Chipotle Aioli
- Classic Caesar
- Country Buttermilk Ranch
- Dijon Balsamic Dressing
- Habanero Salsa
- Honey Mustard
- Horseradish Mayo
- Hot Wing Sauce
- Lemon Vinaigrette
- Mayo
- Red relish
- Roasted garlic aioli
- Russian Dressing
- Tzatziki sauce

In a Bowl

- Lettuce Blend
- Organic Mixed Greens
- Baby Spinach

Shakes and Malts

- Vanilla Shake
- Chocolate Shake
- Peanut Butter Shake
- Banana Shake
- Butterscotch Shake
- Cherry Shake
- Whipped Marshmallow Shake

- Dessert
- Ice cream

The Varsity

Entrees

- Plain Hamburger without the bun and mayonnaise, but with lettuce and tomato
- Grilled Chicken without the bun

Salads

- Garden Salad with any dressing

Shakes

- Frosted Orange Shake
- Chocolate Shake

Wendy's

Entrée

- Hamburger Patty
- Ultimate Chicken Grill Fillet

Baked Potatoes

- Plain
- Sour Cream & Chives
- Cheese
- Bacon & Cheese

- Broccoli & Cheese
- Chili & Cheese

Side Items

- Apple Slices
- Chili
- Hot Chili Seasoning Packet
- Cheddar Cheese, shredded

Frosty™

- Chocolate Frosty
- Vanilla Frosty
- Chocolate Frosty Shake
- Strawberry Frosty Shake
- Vanilla Bean Frosty Shake
- Wild Berry Frosty Shake
- Caramel Frosty Shake
- Caramel Apple Frosty Parfait (without granola)

Salads

- Caesar Side Salad (without croutons)
- Garden Side Salad (without croutons)
- Baja Salad
- Seasoned Tortilla Strips+
- Apple Pecan Chicken Salad (without pecans)
- BLT Cobb Salad

Dressings

- Avocado Ranch Dressing
- Classic Ranch Dressing
- Creamy Red Jalapeno Dressing
- Fat Free French Dressing

- Italian Vinaigrette Dressing
- Lemon Garlic Caesar Dressing
- Light Classic Ranch Dressing
- Pomegranate Vinaigrette Dressing
- Thousand Island Dressing

Sauce and Condiments

- American Cheese
- Applewood Smoked Bacon
- Buttery Best Spread
- Cheddar Cheese Sauce
- Dill Pickles
- Honey Mustard Sauce
- Ketchup
- Lettuce
- Mustard
- Mayonnaise
- Natural Asiago Cheese
- Cheddar & Pepper Jack Cheese Blend
- Red Onion
- Ranch Sauce
- Reduced Fat Sour Cream+
- Tomato
- Tartar Sauce

White Castle

Burgers

Cross contamination does exist. Celiacs or allergenics, do not eat.

- Hamburger patty without the bun

Slider Toppings

- American Cheese
- Jalapeno Cheese
- Bacon (1 slice)
- Bacon Topping

Hamburger Sauce

- Ketchup
- Mustard
- Spicy Hamburger Sauce

Oatmeal

Not *100% safe for Celiacs so beware.*

- Maple and Brown Sugar Oatmeal (w/ Berry Blend Toppings or Honey Roasted Almond Topping)

French Fries

These fries are cooked in common fryers with foods that contain gluten so this is not recommended for anyone with an allergy or Celiac.

- French Fries
- Cheese Fries
- Loaded Fries

Sauces and Condiments

- BBQ Sauce
- Cheese Sauce
- Marinara Sauce
- Ranch
- Seafood Sauce
- Seafood Cocktail Sauce
- White Castle Zesty Zing
- Tartar Sauce

- Apple Sauce
- Fat Free Honey Mustard sauce
- Hot Sauce
- Horseradish Mustard

Crave Coolers

- Coke
- Fanta Wild Cherry

Milkshakes

- Chocolate
- Strawberry
- Vanilla

Wienerschnitzel

Fries

- French Fries
- Chili Cheese Fries

Breakfast

- Breakfast Platter with Bacon
- Breakfast Platter with Sausage
- Hash Browns
- Syrup

Sauces

- Ranch Dressing
- Wing Sauce

Tastee-Freez Desserts

- Old Fashion Sundae: Hot Fudge, Chocolate, Strawberry, Pineapple
- Banana Split
- Milkshakes: Vanilla, Chocolate, Strawberry
- Freezee: M&M's, Butterfinger, Reese's
- Mug Root Beer Float
- Mini Sundae: Hot Fudge, Chocolate, Strawberry

Chicken

Now, I don't want to get your hopes too high on this section because if it's gluten free fried chicken you seek, you'll be disappointed. However, you can still enjoy some tender, juicy grilled chicken from a select number of chicken joints.

Bojangles

Salad

- Garden Salad
- Grilled Chicken Salad

Chicken

- Roasted Chicken Bites

Sides

- Bo-Tato Rounds
- Bojangles Cajun Pintos
- Seasoned Fries
- Picnic Grits
- Green Beans
- Cole Slaw
- Bojangles Dirty Rice

Sauces

- All sauces and dressings

Chick Fil A

Entree

- Chick-fil-A® Chargrilled Chicken Filet
- Chick-fil-A® Grilled nuggets or strips

Salads

- Grilled Market Salad with grilled chicken
- Asian Salad with Grilled Nuggets and no wonton strips
- Cobb Salad with grilled chicken (breaded chicken is standard, so be sure to request grilled chicken) and no dried spicy peppers

Sides

- Fruit Cup
- Side Salad
- Cole Slaw
- Carrot & Raisin Salad
- Chick-fil-A Waffle Potato Fries®
- Yogurt Parfait

Breakfast

- Bacon strips
- Egg
- Sausage patty
- American cheese slice
- Hash Browns

Desserts

- Icedream®
- Milkshakes (Vanilla, Chocolate, and Strawberry)
- Chocolate Syrup

Dipping Sauces and Dressings

- Avocado Lime Ranch
- Zesty Apple Cider Vinaigrette
- Barbecue Sauce
- Honey Mustard Sauce
- Honey Roasted BBQ Sauce
- Polynesian Sauce
- Buttermilk Ranch Sauce
- Chick-fil-A® Buffalo Sauce
- Spicy Dressing
- Buttermilk Ranch Dressing
- Thousand Island Dressing
- Light Italian Dressing
- Fat Free Dijon Honey Mustard Dressing
- Caesar Dressing
- Reduced Fat Raspberry Vinaigrette Dressing
- Reduced Fat Berry Balsamic Vinaigrette Dressing
- Chick-fil-A® Sauce

Chicken Express

Fish

- Catfish

Sides

- Seasoned Italian Green Beans
- Corn on the Cob
- Coleslaw

Desserts

- Chocolate Soft Serve

- Vanilla Soft Serve

Dessert Add Ins

- Caramel
- Heath
- Butterfinger
- Heath
- M&Ms
- Strawberry
- Strawberry Banana
- Mango
- Peach

Sauces

- All sauces

Church's Chicken

Sides

- Corn
- Jalapenos Peppers
- Coleslaw
- Collard Greens
- French Fries
- Cajun Rice

Sauces

- Creamy Jalapeno
- BBQ
- Honey Mustard
- Sweet and Sour

- Ranch
- Ketchup
- Hot Sauce
- Tartar Sauce
- Cocktail Sauce

Kentucky Fried Chicken (KFC)

Because the flour at KFC is airborne, this is NOT a safe place for Celiacs or anyone with a gluten allergy/sensitivity.

Sides

- Three bean salad
- House Side Salad without Dressing
- Green beans
- Corn on the Cobb
- Sweet Cornel Corn
- Potato Salad
- Sargento Light String Cheese

Dipping sauce and Dressings

- Honey Barbeque Sandwich Sauce
- Honey Mustard BBQ Sauce
- Pepper Mayonnaise
- Spicy Mayonnaise
- KFC Signature Sauce Dipping Cup
- Spicy Chipotle Dipping Sauce
- Creamy Ranch Dipping Sauce
- HBBQ Dipping Sauce
- Tartar Sauce
- Honey Sauce
- Colonel's Buttery Spread
- Heinz Buttermilk Ranch Dressing

- Hidden Valley The Original Ranch Fat Free Dressing
- Marzetti Light Italian Dressing

Popeyes

Just like KFC, because the flour at KFC is airborne, this is NOT a safe place for Celiacs or anyone with a gluten allergy/sensitivity.

- Red beans
- Cole slaw
- Corn on the cob (at participating locations)
- Cajun rice

Raising Canes

Entrees

- Chicken Fingers without breading aka "Naked" Chicken Fingers

Sides

- Cole Slaw
- Fries (50/50 – French fries may or may not share the same fryer as the original fried chicken strips with batter)

Sauces and Condiments

- Cane's Sauce

Wingstop

Regular Wings

- Atomic
- Cajun
- Garlic Parmesan
- Hawaiian Renfro
- Hickory Smoked BBQ Ken's
- Hickory Smoked BBQ Refro
- Lemon Pepper
- Louisiana Rub
- Mild
- Original Hot
- Teriyaki Renfro

Sides

- Bourbon Baked Beans
- Coleslaw
- Honey Mustard
- Hot Cheddar Cheese Sauce
- Potato Salad
- Ranch
- Seasoned Fries
- Veggie Sticks (Carrots or Celery)

Zaxby's

Entrees

- Chicken Wings
- The Caesar Zalad with no chicken and no croutons

Sides

- Side Salad
- Cole Slaw
- Crinkle Fries
- Celery
- Tater Chips

Sauces and Dressings

- Thousand Island Dressing
- BBQ Sauce
- Blue Cheese Dressing
- Roadhouse Dressing
- Caesar Dressing
- Honey French Dressing
- Hot Honey Mustard Sauce
- Tongue Torch sauce
- Insane Sauce
- Zax Sauce
- Ketchup
- Lite Ranch Dressing
- Mediterranean Dressing
- Nuclear Sauce
- Original Wing Sauce
- Wimpy Sauce
- Zestable Sauce
- Zax Sauce

Milkshakes

- Chocolate
- Birthday Cake
- Strawberry
- Vanilla

Contemporary & Traditional American

This section is perfect for anyone looking for a
contemporary, more traditional dining experience.

Boston Market

Entrée

- Roasted Turkey Breast
- Rotisserie Chicken

Sides

- Butternut Squash
- Cinnamon Apples
- Coleslaw
- Creamed Spinach
- Fresh Steamed Vegetables
- Garlic Dill New Potatoes
- Mashed Potatoes
- Sweet Corn
- Loaded Mashed Potatoes
- Mediterranean Green Beans
- Garlicky Spinach

Salads

- Southwest Santa Fe

Sauces

- Frank's Sweet Heat
- Honey Habanero
- Island Mojo

Burtons Grill

Be sure to request the gluten free lunch and dinner menu, as seen below.

Appetizers

- Baked Stuffed Zucchini
- Buffalo Chicken Dip
- Spicy Calamari
- Spinach and Artichoke Dip

Salads

- Chopped Blue Cheese Salad
- Caesar Salad
- House Salad
- Marinated Mediterranean Salad
- Harvest Salad
- BBQ Chicken Salad
- Steakhouse Salad
- Beet Salad

Sandwiches and Burgers

- Classic Cheeseburger
- Maxx Burger
- Pacific Coast Burger
- Haddock Sandwich
- Steak Sandwich

Chef Specials

- Mediterranean Chicken
- Salmon Piccata
- Risotto of the Day
- Short Rib Sherpherd's Pie

- Salmon
- Burtons Classics
- Shrimp Scampi
- Lobster and Shrimp Pasta
- Scallop Risotto
- Salmon Piccata

Land and Sea

- Braised Short Ribs
- Chicken and Wild Mushroom Pasta
- Chicken Duo

Desserts

- Vanilla Bean Creme Brulee
- Warmed Chocolate Torte
- Vanilla Ice Cream
- Sorbet

Cocktails

- Distilled Spirits
- Wine
- Redbridge Beer

Chart House

Appetizers

- Crab, Avocado Mango Stack
- Hummus Trio
- Jumbo Shrimp Cocktail
- Oyster on ½ Shell
- Herb Steam Artichoke

Salads

- Chicken Cobb Salad
- Seafood Cobb Salad
- Chopped Spinach Salad
- Caesar Salad
- Chart House Chopped Salad

Seafood

- King Crab
- Live Maine Lobster
- Lobster Tail
- Today's Fresh Fish
- Mahi
- Salmon
- Swordfish
- Ahi Tuna
- Tilapia
- Grouper
- White Sea Bass
- Snapper
- Halibut
- Signature Fish
- Bronze Fresh Fish
- Fresh Fish Del Mar

Steaks, Poultry, Prime Rib

- New Wave Surf & Turf
- Grilled Chicken
- Prime Rib
- Oscar Medallions
- Short Ribs
- Filet Mignon
- NY Shrimp
- Prime Rib & Grilled Shrimp

- Filet & Shrimp

Desserts

- Crème Brulee
- Raspberry Sorbetini

Claim Jumper

Salads

- California Citrus Chicken Salad without bleu cheese crumbles
- BBQ Chicken Salad

Entrees

- Rotisserie Chicken
- Norwegian Salmon
- Giant Stuffed Baker: No Alfredo sauce
- BBQ Baby Back Pork Ribs
- California Chicken Tortillas
- Ribs & Chicken
- Grilled Steaks & Lobster
- Top Sirloin
- Filet Mignon
- Ribeye Steak
- New York Strip
- Porterhouse Steak
- Top Sirloin & Lobster Tail
- Filet Mignon & Lobster Tail
- Chopped Steak
- Claim Jumper K-Bob without rice pilaf

Crave

Be sure to request the gluten free menu before you order.

Appetizers

- Crave Wings
- Chipotle BBQ Baby Back Ribs
- Edamame
- Mediterranean Plate
- Chilled Shrimp and Butternut Carpaccio

Soups and Starter Salads

Be sure to order the salads without croutons

- Hearty Tomato Pesto
- Crave Salad
- Grilled Caesar Salad
- Poached Pear and Goat Cheese Salad

Entrée Salads

- Black and Bleu Steak Salad
- Grilled Salmon Salad

Brick Oven Specialties

- Double Cut Pork Chop
- Roasted Salmon with Cranberry Bacon Crust

From the Grill

- Flat Iron Steak
- Grilled Rib Eye Steak
- Mixed Vegetable Grill
- Grilled Atlantic Salmon

Franklin Café

- Roasted Rutabaga Bisque
- Arugula Salad
- Little Gem Salad
- Skillet Smoked Mussels
- Cherry Wood Roasted Beets
- Beef Tartare
- Grilled Shrimp
- Steak Frites
- Braised Short Rib

Houlihan's

Appetizers and Shareables

- Steamed Edamame without the shaoxing sauce
- Side Salad
- House Salad without croutons (select balsamic vinaigrette as your dressing)

Entrees

- Premium Steaks (request that vegetables be cooked in olive oil and seasoned with salt & pepper only)
- 8 oz Filet Mignon
- 12 oz New York Strip
- 9 oz USDA Prime Top Sirloin
- Grilled 4 oz Petite Filet Mignon (request that vegetables be cooked in olive oil or butter and seasoned with salt & pepper only)
- BBQ Baby Back Ribs with today's vegetables and french fries
- Fire Grilled Atlantic Salmon (request that vegetables be cooked in olive oil and seasoned with salt & pepper only)

Entree Salads

- Heartland Grilled Chicken Salad without croutons and focaccia roll
- Spinach Salad with Grilled Chicken without foccacia roll
- Handhelds
- Creekstone Farms Black Angus Burger ordered without the bun
- Brentwood Chicken Sandwich ordered without the bun

Sides

- Honest Gold Mashed Potatoes
- Tortilla Chips and Homemade Salsa
- Today's Vegetables (request with olive oil and salt & pepper only)
- Baked Potato
- French Fries

Dessert

- Creme Brûlée

Jack's Family Restaurant

Breakfast

- Hashbrowns

Breakfast Sides

- Mashed Potatoes (with or without butter)
- Green beans
- Coleslaw
- Sausage
- Bacon

- Steak
- Bologna
- Ham
- Pork Chop
- Egg

Lunch

- Grilled Chicken Platter

Salads without Dressing and Croutons

- Side Salad
- Side Salad without Cheese
- Spring Salad
- Grilled Chicken Salad

Sandwiches

- Hamburger Patty

Fries

- All fries

Desserts

- Chocolate Peanut Butter Ice Cream (or milkshake)
- Butter Crunch Ice Cream (or milkshake)
- Orange Sherbet (or milkshake)
- Strawberry Ice Cream (or milkshake)
- Buttered Pecan Ice Cream (or milkshake)
- Vanilla Ice Cream (or milkshake)

Joey Restaurants

Entrées and Starters

- Steamed Edamame
- Sashimi Tuna Salad
- Beach Salad
- Lunch Salmon
- Dinner Salmon

Steaks

- Cab Top Sirloin
- Filet Mignon
- Cab New York
- Steak and Prawns

Max and Erma's

Munchies aka Appetizers

- Wings
- Potato Skins
- Chips and Salsa: with corn tortilla chips
- Grilled Asparagus

Salads

- House Garden Salad: No croutons or breadstick
- Baby Green Salads: No croutons or breadstick
- Third Street Salad: No croutons or breadstick
- Caesar Salad: No croutons or breadstick
- Chicken Caesar Salad: No croutons or breadstick
- Santa Fe Salad: No tortilla strips or breadstick
- Apple Pecan Salad: No breadstick

Specialties

- Laredo Steak
- Max's Sirloin
- Classic Sirloin
- Grilled Chicken
- Salmon
- Spicy Cajun Tilapia

Sides

- Fruit Salad
- Asparagus
- Applesauce
- Cole Slaw
- Broccoli

Fresh Seasonal Vegetables

Just for the Pups aka Kids' Menu

- Grilled Chicken with Broccoli
- Kids Sliders No Bun: served with fruit salad

The Melting Pot

Cheese Fondue

- Spinach Artichoke Cheese Fondue: Request to be made with cornstarch
- Fiesta Cheese Fondue: Request to be made with cornstarch and Redbridge beer
- Cheddar Cheese Fondue: Request to be made with Redbridge beer and no Worcestershire sauce

- Wisconsin Trio Cheese Fondue: Request to be make with cornstarch
- Traditional Swiss Cheese Fondue: Request to be made with cornstarch

Gluten-Free Salads

- The Melting Pot House Salad: Request no crotons
- Spinach Mushroom Salad
- Caesar Salad: Request no croutons
- California Salad

Gluten-Free Entrées

- Land & Sea
- The French Quarter
- Seafood Trio
- All Natural Breast of Chicken
- Cedar Plank Salmon
- Pacific Rim
- The Vegetarian
- Filet Mignon

Entrée Cooking Styles

- Coq au Vin
- Court Bouillon
- Bourguignonne: Request no batters
- Mojo

Entrée Sauces

- Curry
- Green Goddess
- Gorgonzola Port
- Ginger Plum

Gluten-Free Chocolate Fondue

- The Original
- Yin & Yang
- Flaming Turtle
- Pure Chocolate
- Bananas Foster
- Chocolate S'mores
- Special Event
- Cookies 'n Cream Marshmallow Dream: Request no Oreo cookies

99 Restaurants

Salads

- Caesar Salad without croutons and Rustic Bread
- Chicken Caesar Salad without croutons and Rustic Bread
- Garden Salad
- Dressings: Buttermilk Ranch, Honey Mustard, Northern Italian

Burgers

All burgers are served with a Gluten-Free Roll

- All Star Burger
- Bacon & Cheese Burger

Entrees

- Broiled Sirloin Tips
- Smothered Tips
- Balsamic Grilled Chicken

- Seasoned Salmon
- Herbed Salmon and Vegetables
- Prime Rib
- NY Strip Sirloin

Kids' Menu

- Junior Top Sirloin Steak
- Junior Burger with Cheese: Specify Gluten-Free Roll

Sides

- Garlic Red Skin Mashed Potatoes
- Baked Potato
- Toppings: Cheese, Bacon and Chives
- Broccoli
- Miss Vickie's Simple Sea Salt Potato Chips
- Motts Natural Applesauce

Desserts

- Hot Fudge Sundae

O'Charley's

Salads

- California Chicken Salad without dressing
- Cedar Planked Tilapia
- Chicken Apple Spinach Salad with Dressing
- Classic Bleu Cheese Wedge

Salad Dressings

- Balsamic Vinaigrette
- Bleu Cheese

- Caesar
- Honey Mustard
- Honey Apple Cider Vinaigrette
- Light Ranch
- Oil & Red Wine Vinegar
- Oil & Vinegar
- Ranch
- Thousand Island

Entrées

- Grilled Atlantic Salmon
- Grilled Top Sirloin
- Jr. Grilled Chicken
- Jr. Grilled Steak
- Louisiana Sirloin
- O'Charley's Baby Back Ribs
- Steak and Grilled Atlantic Salmon
- Steak and Half-Rack Baby Back Ribs
- Your Favorite Rib Eye Steak

Soup

- Cream of Tomato Basil
- Overloaded Potato
- Roasted Poblano Chowder

Sides

- Asparagus
- Baked Potato (loaded or plain)
- With whipped butter
- With Sour cream
- Bleu Cheese Steak Topping
- Broccoli a la carter
- Eggs
- Smashed Potatoes

- Sautéed Onions
- Southern Slaw

Seasons 52

Appetizers

- Edamame
- Spicy Tuna Roll

Salads

- Mixed Green Salad
- Baby Spinach Salad
- Kalymnos Greek Salad

Entrees

- Grilled Boneless Rainbow trout without vegetable glaze
- Cedar Plank Atlantic Salmon
- Wood Roasted Pork Tenderloin without sherry glaze
- Grilled Rack of New Zealand Lamb without Dijon sauce

Sandwiches without Bun Accompanied by Fresh Green Salad

- Turkey Burger without Dijon mustard
- Blackened Fish
- Western Buffalo Burger

Desserts

- Fresh Seasonal Fruit Mini

Village Tavern

Be sure to let your server know that you will be ordering off their gluten free menu.

Appetizer Salads

- Spinach
- Garden without croutons
- Tavern Salad

Large Salads

- Grilled Chicken Spinach
- Greek Salad
- Tavern House Salad

Salad Dressings

- Basil Vinaigrette
- Balsamic Vinaigrette,
- Tavern Vinaigrette
- Whole Grain Mustard and Honey
- Poppyseed
- Thousand Island
- Ranch

Fish Market Fresh Fish

- Grilled Tilapia
- Grilled Salmon
- Grouper Hemingway

Steakhouse Steaks and Prime Rib

- Filet Mignon
- Ribeye
- Top Sirloin

- New York Strip

Tavern Specialties

- Spaghetti Squash and Zucchini
- Maple Cured Pork
- Pan Seared Scallops

Sides

- Sautéed Vegetables
- Garlic Mashed Potatoes
- Green Beans
- Loaded Baked Potato
- Asparagus
- Sautéed Spinach

Desserts

- Raspberry Sorbet
- Creme Brulee

Desserts, Drinks, & Coffee

Do you have a craving for something sweet and delicious?
Do you need a caffeine boost? Or are you addicted to all
things sweet and delicious? If so, this is your section.

Baskin Robbins

Hand Scooped

- Premium Churned Light Cappuccino Chip
- Premium Churned Reduced Fat, No Sugar Added
  Caramel Truffle Turtle
- Super Soldier Swirl
- Firehouse
- Toffee Pecan Crunch
- White Caramel Chocolate Frozen Yogurt
- Fat Free Vanilla Frozen Yogurt
- Watermelon Chip
- Pink Grapefruit Sorbet
- Premium Churned Reduced Fat Pineapple Coconut
- Premium Churned Reduced Chocolate Overload
- Premium Churned Reduced Butter Almond Crunch
- Tax Crunch®
- Cotton Candy
- Jamoca®
- Mint Chocolate Chip
- Jamoca® Almond Fudge
- Mint Chocolate Chip
- Jamoca® Almond Fudge
- Lemon Custard
- Pistachio Almond
- Oregon Black Berry
- Baseball Nut®

- Pumpkin Pie
- Egg Nog
- Nutty Coconut
- Bananas 'n Strawberries
- Pralines 'n Cream
- Quarterback Crunch®
- Gold Medal Ribbon
- Banana Nut
- Chocolate Mousse Royal®
- Cherries Jubilee
- World Class® Chocolate
- Winter White Chocolate®
- Reese's® Peanut Butter Cup
- Snickers®
- Chocolate
- Peanut Butter 'n Chocolate
- Chocolate Chip
- Very Berry Strawberry
- Rum Raisin
- Chocolate Almond
- Vanilla
- Old Fashioned Butter Pecan
- Love Potion #31®
- Creole Cream Cheese
- Chocolate Fudge
- Orange Sherbet
- Rock 'n Pop Swirl
- Wild 'n Reckless Sherbet
- Splish Splash® Sherbet
- Rainbow Sherbet
- Daiquiri Ice
- Lemon Sorbet
- Tropical Ice
- Watermelon Chip

Soft Serve

- Strawberry Fruit Cream
- Peach Passion Fruit Cream
- Reese's® Mini Parfait
- Strawberry 'n Almonds
- Vanilla
- Reese's® Peanut Butter Cup
- Heath® 31°
- Strawberry Banana Below 31°
- Mango Fruit Cream
- Hot Fudge Sundae
- Strawberry
- Caramel Sundae
- Butterfinger®
- Jamoca® Almond Fudge

Sundaes

- Two-scoop
- Classic Banana Split
- Banana Royale
- Reese's® Peanut Butter Cup
- Snickers®

Beverages

- Cappuccino Blast® Nonfat
- Freeze with Orange Sherbet
- Ice Cream Soda with Vanilla
- Ice Cream Float with Vanilla and Root Beer
- Chocolate Chip Shake
- Peach Passion Banana Fruit Blast Smoothie
- Peach Passion Fruit Blast
- Raspberry Chip Shake with premium Churned Light Raspberry Chip ice cream
- Chocolate Shake

- Strawberry Banana Fruit Blast Smoothie
- Strawberry Citrus Fruit Blast
- Cappuccino Blast® Original
- Cappuccino Blast® Nonfat
- Cappuccino Blast® Mocha
- Vanilla Shake
- Chocolate Shake with Vanilla ice cream
- Chocolate Shake with Chocolate ice cream
- Cappuccino Blast® Turtle
- Wild Mango Fruit Blast
- Strawberry Shake
- Wild Mango Fruit Blast
- Mango Fruit Blast Smoothie
- Cappuccino Blast® Original
- Mint Chocolate Chip Shake
- Cappuccino Blast® Caramel
- Cappuccino Blast® with Soft Serve

Brooklyn Ice Cream Factory

Ice Cream

- Vanilla
- Strawberry
- Vanilla Chocolate Chunk
- Chocolate Chocolate Chunk
- Peaches & Cream
- Butter Pecan
- Coffee

Carvel

Ice Cream and Sherbet

- Chocolate Ice Cream
- Lemon Sherbet Flavor
- Lime Sherbet Flavor
- Low Fat Chocolate Ice Cream
- Low Fat Vanilla Ice Cream
- No Sugar Added Vanilla Ice Cream
- Orange Sherbet Flavor
- Vanilla Ice Cream

Toppings and Syrups

- Almonds, diced
- Banana Pudding (used to make banana ice cream)
- Bittersweet Fudge
- Black Bordeaux Cherries
- Black Raspberry Puree
- Brown Bonnet
- Butter Flavor
- Butterfinger, ground
- Butterscotch Topping
- Caramel Fudge Topping
- Carvella Flavor
- Cheesecake Base Flavor
- Cherry Bonnet
- Chocolate Chips
- Chocolate Pieces
- Chocolate Pre-Pak
- Chocolate Sprinkles
- Chocolate Syrup
- Citric Acid
- Coconut, toasted
- Coconut, white

- Coffee Flavor
- Confetti Sprinkles
- Edible Images
- Egg Nog Base
- Heath Bar, ground
- Maple Flavor
- Maraschino Cherries, ½'s
- Maraschino Cherries, whole
- Marshmallow Topping
- Milk Fudge
- Mini M&M's
- Mint Flavor
- Peaches, diced
- Peanut Butter Topping
- Peanuts, granulated
- Pecans, chopped
- Pineapple Cubes
- Piping Gel
- Pistachio Flavor
- Praline Pecans
- Pumpkin Puree
- Rainbow, Sprinkles
- Reese's Peanut Butter Cup, ground
- Reese's Pieces
- Rum Flavor
- Sherbet
- Simple Syrup
- Strawberries
- Strawberry Pre-Pak
- Strawberry Puree
- Walnuts, chopped
- Whipped Cream
- White Bonnet

Cold Stone Creamery

Since there's a high chance of cross contamination if your ice cream is mixed on the "cold stone," just be sure to let your the workers know that you have an allergy so that they clean the "cold stone" mixing plate properly.

Ice Cream

- Amaretto
- Banana
- Butter Pecan
- Candy Cane
- Cheesecake
- Chocolate Dipped Strawberry
- Chocolate
- Chocolate Hazelnut
- Chocolate Peanut Butter Cup
- Cinnamon
- Coconut
- Coffee
- Cotton Candy
- Dark Chocolate
- Dark Chocolate Peppermint
- Egg Nog
- French Toast
- French Vanilla
- Ghirardelli Chocolate
- Irish Cream
- Key Lime
- Macadamia Nut
- Mango
- Marshmallow
- Mint
- Mocha
- Orange Dreamsicle

- Peanut Butter
- Pecan Praline
- Pistachio
- Pumpkin
- Raspberry
- Salted Caramel
- Sinless Sans Fat Free Sweet Cream
- Strawberry
- Sweet Cream
- Vanilla Bean
- White Chocolate

Sorbet and Yogurt

- Country Time Lemonade Sorbet
- Lemon Sorbet
- Strawberry Mango Banana Sorbet
- Pineapple Orange Banana Sorbet
- Raspberry Sorbet
- Watermolon Sorbet
- Chocolate Yogurt
- Raspberry Yogurt
- Salt and Caramel Yogurt
- Vanilla Yogurt
- Smoothies
- Lemon Ice
- Mango
- Orange Juice
- Lifestyle Smoothie Mix

Mix-Ins

- Butterfinger
- HEATH
- M&Ms
- Peanut M&Ms
- REESE'S Peanut Butter Cup

- SNICKERS Candy
- ALMOND JOY Candy
- REESE'S Pieces
- YORK Peppermint Patties
- Chocolate Chips
- Chocolate Shavings
- Gummi Bears
- White Chocolate Chips
- Rainbow Sprinkles
- Chocolate Sprinkles
- Coconut
- Gumballs
- Fruit
- Apple Pie Filling
- Bananas
- Black Cherries
- Blackberries
- Blueberries
- Cherry Pie Filling
- Maraschino Cherries
- Peach Pie Filing
- Pineapple Tidbits
- Raisins
- Raspberries
- Strawberries
- Toppings
- Butterscotch Fat Free
- Caramel Fat Free
- Caramel
- Cinnamon
- Fudge Fat Free
- Fudge
- Honey
- Marshmallow Creme
- Redi Wip Original
- Whipped Topping

- Nuts
- Cashews
- Macadamia Nuts
- Peanuts
- Pecan Pralines
- Pecans
- Pistachios
- Roasted Almonds
- Sliced Almonds
- Walnuts

Dunkin Donuts

- Gluten free muffins and donuts (in select locations)
- All coffee
- All beverages

Haagen Dazs

Haagen Dazs Ice Cream

- Butter Pecan
- Cherry Vanilla
- Chocolate
- Chocolate Chocolate Chip
- Chocolate Peanut Butter
- Coffee
- Creme Brulee
- Dark Chocolate
- Dulce De Leche
- Green Tea
- Java Chip

- Mango
- Mint Chip
- Pineapple Coconut
- Pistachio
- Rocky Road
- Rum Raisin
- Strawberry
- Vanilla
- Vanilla Bean
- Vanilla Chocolate Chip
- Vanilla Swiss Almond
- White Chocolate Raspberry Truffle

Haagen Dazs Five Ice Cream

- Coffee
- Lemon
- Milk Chocolate
- Vanilla Bean

Haagen Dazs Limited Edition Ice Cream

- Vanilla Bean Espresso
- Salted Caramel Truffle
- Peppermint Bark

Haagen Dazs Sorbet

- Blackberry Cabernet
- Chocolate
- Mango
- Orchard Peach
- Rspberry
- Strawberry
- Zesty Lemon

Haagen Dazs Ice Cream & Sorbet Cups

- Chocolate
- Chocolate Peanut Butter
- Coffee
- Dulce De Leche
- Mango Sorbet
- Raspberry Sorbet
- Rum Raisin
- Strawberry Vanilla

Haagen Dazs Low Fat Frozen Yogurt

- Coffee
- Vanilla
- Vanilla Raspberry Swirl

Haagen Dazs Ice Cream Bars

- Chocolate Dark Chocolate
- Raspberry and Vanilla Milk Chocolate
- Vanilla Dark Chocolate
- Vanilla Milk Chocolate
- Vanilla Milk Chocolate Almond
- Vanilla and Raspberry Swirl
- Salted Caramel 3 Pack
- Peppermint Bark 3 Pack
- Chocolate Dark Chocolate Bars
- Coffee Almond Crunch Bars
- Vanilla Milk Chocolate Bars
- Vanilla Milk Chocolate Almond Bars
- Raspberry and Vanilla Milk Chocolate Bars
- Coffee Almond Crunch
- Vanilla Chocolate Almond

Jamba Juice

Drinks and Smoothies

- 3G Charger Boost
- Acai Super-Antioxidant
- Antioxidant Power Boost
- Apple 'n Greens
- Banana Berry
- Berry Fulfilling
- Berry UpBeet
- Blackberry Bliss
- Caribbean Passion
- Carrot Juice
- Chocolate Moo'd
- Classic Hot Chocolate
- Coffee Craze
- Five Fruit Frenzy
- Flax and Fiber Boost
- Immunity Boost
- Mango Mantra
- Mango-a-go-go
- Matcha Energy Shot-Orange Juice
- Matcha Energy Shot-Soymilk
- Matcha Green Tea Blast
- Mega Mango
- Mocha Mojo
- Orange Carrot Karma
- Orange Dream Machine
- Orange Juice
- Orange-A-Peel
- Organic African Nectar
- Organic Breakfast
- Organic Detox Infusion
- Organic Earl Grey
- Organic Green Drago

- Organic House Blend
- Organic House Blend Decaf
- Organic Spring Jasmine
- Original Spiced Chai
- Peach Perfection
- Peach Pleasure
- Peanut Butter Moo'd
- Pomegranate Paradise
- Pomegranate Pick-Me-Up
- Protein Berry Workout
- Pumpkin Smash
- Razzmatazz
- Soy Protein Boost
- Strawberries Wild
- Strawberry Nirvana
- Strawberry Surf Rider
- Strawberry Whirl
- The Coldbuster
- Whey Protein Boost

Orange Julius

Premium Light Smoothies

- Strawberry Banana
- Mango Pineapple
- Tripleberry
- Pina Colada
- Berry-Pom
- OrangeBerry
- Orange
- Strawberry

Light Smoothies

- Strawberry Banana
- Mango Pineapple
- Pina Colada
- Berry-Pom
- OrangeBerry
- Orange
- Strawberry

Julius Originals

- Strawberry Banana
- Mango Pineapple
- Tripleberry
- Pina Colada
- Berry-Pom
- OrangeBerry
- Orange
- Strawberry

Pinkberry

Unfortunately, no frozen yogurts are gluten free.

Fresh Yogurt

- Greek Yogurt

Toppings

- all natural mixed nuts
- almond roca
- caramelized almonds
- carob chips

- chocolate chips
- coconut
- nutella
- nutmeg
- organic chili powder
- organic fruity bears
- organic strawberry jam
- roasted hazelnuts
- sea salt
- shaved milk chocolate
- toasted almond
- white chocolate shavings
- yogurt chips

Red Mango

All frozen yogurt flavors are gluten free, however, please be careful with the toppings since some of them may contain traces of wheat, gluten, nuts, etc.

- All natural frozen yogurt
- All frozen coffee chillers
- All frozen lemonades
- All sorbettos

Starbucks

Be sure to tell your barista that you have a gluten allergy so that they take the proper precautions to limit any cross contamination. You don't want to get a coffee that somehow got contaminated with the vanilla bean powder (has gluten). Also, watch out for the Skinny Vanilla Latte.

Salads

- Deluxe Fruit Blend

Yogurt Parfaits

- Dark Cherry Yogurt Parfait
- Strawberry and Blueberry Yogurt Parfait
- Greek Yogurt Parfait

Drinks and Beverages

- Starbucks DoubleShot Energy+…all flavors
- Starbucks Bottled Frappucino Coffee Drink…all flavors
- Bold Pick of the Day
- Café Misto
- Clover Brewed Coffee
- Coffee Traveler
- Decaf Pike Place Roast
- Iced Coffee
- Iced Coffee with Milk
- Pike Place Roast
- Hot Chocolate
- Peppermint Hot Chocolate
- Salted Caramel Hot Chocolate
- White Hot Chocolate
- All Espresso
- All Vivanno Smoothies
- All Tazo Teas EXCEPT: Green Ginger, Tazo Honeybush, Lemon Ginger, and Tea Lemonade
- All Kid's Drinks

Frappuccino Blended Beverages

- Café Vanilla
- Caramel
- Caramel Brulee

- Cinnamon Dolce
- Cinnamon Crème
- Coconut Crème
- Coffee
- Espresso
- Extra Coffee
- Mocha Coconut
- Mocha
- Java Chip
- Peppermint Mocha
- Soy Strawberries Crème (Starbucks uses Eden organic soy milk, so if ordering something soy you need to ask which version they are using. The unsweetened does not contain gluten, but the original does so watch out)
- Tazo Chai Crème
- Tazo Green Teal Crème
- White Chocolate Crème
- White Chocolate Mocha

TCBY

Soft Serve

- Vanilla
- Chocolate
- Classic Tart
- Dutch Chocolate
- Coffee
- Strawberry
- Golden Vanilla
- Old Fashioned Vanilla
- Fat Free Mountain Black Berry
- White Chocolate Macadamia Nut
- White Chocolate Mouse

- Mango Sorbet
- Kiwi Strawberry Sorbet
- Orange Sorbet
- Ruby Red Grapefruit Sorbet

Hand Scooped

- Butter pecan Perfection
- Chocolate Chocolate
- Mint Chocolate Chunk
- Cotton Candy
- Mocha Almond
- Peaches and Cream
- Peanut Butter Delight
- Pralines and Cream
- Vanilla Bean
- Vanilla Chocolate Chunk
- Very Berry Strawberry
- White Chocolate Mouse
- Rainbow Cream
- Psychedelic Sorbet

Toppings

- All fruit toppings
- Caramel topping
- Hot fudge topping
- Chocolate topping
- Marshmallow topping
- Whipped topping
- Peanut Butter topping

Family & Breakfast

Don't you just love those restaurants that serve breakfast 24 hours a day? I do. And if you do too, this is the perfect section of gluten free menus for you and your family.

Bob Evan's

Breakfast

Be sure to request no bread, toast, or pancakes (or any other breads)

- The Rise and Shine
- Steak and Farm Fresh Eggs
- The Big Egg Breakfast
- Pot Roast Hash
- All omelets with regular eggs, egg lites, or egg whites
- Turkey Sausage Breakfast
- Sunrise
- The Mini Sampler

A La Carte Sides

- All breakfast meats
- All breakfast sides
- Grits
- Mini fruit and yogurt parfaits

Lunch Items

Be sure to ask for your sandwich to be wrapped in lettuce instead of their bread options.

- The Farm Favorite Burger
- The Three Cheese Burger

- Big Farm Bacon Cheeseburger
- Big Farm Hamburger
- The Farm Favorite Grilled Chicken Sandwich
- Farm Grill Chicken Club
- Farm Grill Chicken Sandwich

Salads

- All dressings
- Apple Cranberry Spinach Salad without pecans
- Cranberry Pecan Chicken Salad without pecans
- Heritage Chef Salad
- Cobb Salad
- Wildfire Chicken Salad with grilled chicken without tortilla strips

Dinner

- Slow Roasted Turkey Breast without gravy, bread, and celery dressing
- Grilled Chicken Breast
- Grilled Chicken Strips
- Salmon Fillet
- Pot Roast without gravy

Signature Soups

- Hearty beef vegetable

Farmhouse Sides

- Applesauce
- Baked russet potato
- Buttered sweet corn
- Seasonal fresh fruit dish
- Glazed fresh baby carrots
- Golden brown home fries

- Shredded hash browns
- Fresh steamed broccoli
- Farmhouse Garden Salad without croutons
- Kid's fresh garden salad without crouton

Kid's Meal

- Fruit dippers
- Lil Farmer's Breakfast without hotcakes
- Sunny Scrambles without toast
- Grilled chicken strip
- Turkey Lurkey without gravy

Dessert

- Vanilla Ice Cream
- Toppings: Chocolate Sauce, Caramel Sauce, Blueberry Topping, Strawberry topping

Dave & Busters

Soups

- Beef Broth
- Chicken Broth

Salads

Be sure to order with no tortilla strips

- Grilled Steak Salad: No frazzled onions
- Honey Mustard Spinach Salad
- House Salad
- Sweep Apple Pecan Salad (Chicken or Shrimp)

Buster's Burgers

Order with no fries and no bun

- Bars Burger
- Buster's Cheeseburger
- Dave's Double Cheeseburger
- Monterey Burger

Chicken & Seafood

- Baked or Grilled Salmon
- Lacy's Chicken
- Plain Grilled Chicken

Grilled Steaks

Request no frazzled onions

- Chargrilled NY Strip
- Chargrilled Sirloin Steak
- NY Strip
- Sirloin Steak

Sides

- Edamame
- Mixed Vegetable Medley
- Sautéed Green Beans

Sauces & Extras

- Guacamole
- Pico de Gallo
- Salsa
- Sour Cream

Kids

- Grilled Chicken
- Kid's Burger: Request no fries and no bun

Denny's

Entrée

- 2 Egg & More Breakfast with Hash Browns with no bread
- Bacons Cheddar Burger Patty with Grapes with no bun
- Beef Patty
- Eggs/Omelets
- Grilled Tilapia: request no rice pilaf
- Sliced/Shaved Ham
- Steak
- Ultimate Omelet with Hash Browns with no bread

Salads

- Side Garden Salad with no croutons dressing

Sides

- Applesauce
- Baby Carrots (raw)
- Black-eyed peas
- Celery Sticks
- Corn
- Fresh Fruit
- Fried Corn Tortilla
- Green Bean
- Hashed Browns
- High Div'n Veggies: No breadsticks, no dip

- Jump-Shot Jello
- Mashed Potatoes
- Olives
- Pinto Beans
- Red Grapes
- Regular French Fries
- Sliced Cucumbers
- Tomato Slices
- Vanilla Yogurt

Sauces

- Lemon Butter Sauce
- Pico de Gallo
- Salsa
- Tartar Sauce

Eat N Park

Breakfast

- All Omelets
- All Scrambler Breakfast Sandwiches (order with gluten free bun)
- Breakfast Combo with no toast
- Breakfast Smile with no toast
- Eggs Breakfast with no toast

Breakfast Sides

- Bacon
- Canadian Bacon
- Fruit Cup
- Home Fries
- Maple Syrup

- Sausage
- Turkey Sausage
- Strawberries
- **Salads and Dressings**
- All Dressings
- Chicken Fajita Salad without tortilla bowl
- Grilled Chicken Salad without french fries
- Steak Salad without french fries
- Taco Salad without tortilla bowl

Burgers

All Black Angus Burgers when ordered with a gluten free bun

Dinner

- Baked Cod without breadcrumbs and seasoning
- Baked Cod Floridian without seasoning
- Beef Liver and Onions
- Rosemary Chicken
- Smothered Ground Sirloin without gravy

Sides

- Applesauce
- Baked Potato
- Bean Medley
- Carrots
- Chili (no crackers)
- Coleslaw
- Corn
- Cottage Cheese
- Fresh Broccoli
- Garden Salad (no croutons)
- Mashed Potatoes (no gravy)
- Sugar Snap Peas

Heath N Kettle

Be sure to tell your server that you have a gluten allergy.

Heart Cape Cod Breakfasts

- Bacon and Eggs
- Flat iron steak and eggs
- Harvest hash and eggs
- Corned beef hash and eggs
- Organic egg white frittata
- Lite and hearty

Country Egg Omelets

- Bacon tomato and cheese
- Baby bella veggie
- Brazilian
- Hash, onion, and cheese
- Steak 'n cheese
- Florentine
- Healthy start

Side Orders

- Fresh fruit
- Bacon
- Harvest hash
- Hash or turkey bacon
- Applewood smoked nitrate free bacon

Appetizers

- Fresh garden salad
- H'nk Signature salads
- H'n K Chili

Early Bird Value Menu

- Grilled liver and onions
- Seafood medley
- Cape scrod

Garden Salad Entrees

- Apple pecan salad
- Organic salad
- Greek salad
- Spinach salad
- Garden salad
- Toppings: grilled chicken, chicken salad, and grilled garlic shrimp

Lunch and Dinner Entrees

Be sure to order sandwiches without bread.

- Bleu Cheese Flat Iron
- Stir Fry Bowls
- Cape Scrod
- Grilled Salmon
- Seafood Medley
- Grilled Flat Iron Steak
- Lemon Ginger Scallops

Foreign, Asian, & International

Do you have a palate for foreign cuisines? If so, in this section you'll find everything from Asian noodles and Chinese fare all the way to Hawaiian fusion and Mediterranean flare.

Kona Grill

Appetizer

- edamame

Salads

Salad dressings: honey dijon, honey balsamic vinaigrette, and oil & vinegar (plus, balsamic, red & white wine vinegar are available

- house salad
- roasted asparagus salad
- kona chopped salad

Burgers without the Bun

- big kahuna cheeseburger without bun
- cheeseburger sliders without bun
- turkey burger

Steaks, Chicken, and Fish

- kona filet
- grilled chicken
- pan-seared ahi
- grilled salmon
- miso-sake marinated sea bass
- grilled fresh fish

Sides

- sautéed baby bok choy
- steamed white rice
- seasonal vegetables

Sushi and Sashimi

- crab
- octopus
- salmon
- shrimp
- sweet shrimp
- tuna
- whitefish

- yellowtail
- whitefish ceviche
- houston roll
- philadelpia roll
- spicy yellowtail roll
- tuna roll

Dessert

- passion fruit creme brûlée

Mama Fu's

Before I get into the menu, I'm just going to let you know that the Mama Fu's gluten free menu is not available in all markets as of yet, but it is soon to be on its way everywhere.

And as another side note, for all Rice Dish and Noodle Bowl entrees, select only Chicken, Shrimp or Veggie.

Okay, so now that we got that out of the way, lets start talking about food.

Appetizers

- Edamame

- Chicken Lettuce Wraps
- Seared Ahi Tuna

Salads

- Garden Side Salad
- Ginger Sesame Salad with Chicken or Peanut Soy Salad with Chicken
- Thai Dynamite Shrimp Salad

Rice Dishes

All fried rice dishes must be prepared with Mama's gluten free sauce

- Sweet N Sour
- Steam Bowl
- Rice Dishes that can be prepared GF: Spicy General Fu Mongolian, Teriyaki Honey Glazed, Sesame Ginger Broccoli, Thai Cashew Stir Fry Orange Peel, Fried Rice

Noodle Bowls

Be sure to request rice noodles and Mama's gluten free sauce. Don't get the tofu on the Thai Pad.

- Lo Mein
- Pad Thai
- Thai Basil
- Singapore Noodles
- Thai Food Noodles

Seared Entrees

- Seared Ahi Tuna Steak

Sides

- Thai Green Bean
- Fried Rice
- Edamame

Kids Selections

- Scooby Fui
- Ninja Noodles
- Mel's Mel's

On a final note, be sure to emphasize that you are ordering off the gluten free menu.

Manchu Wok

Rice & Noodles

- Steamed Rice

Vegetables

- Mixed Vegetables

Noodles & Company

Be sure to order rice noodles with any of the dishes below.

Noodle Entrée

- Pad Thai with rice noodles
- Penne Rosa with rice noodles
- Pasta Fresca with rice noodles

- Whole Grain Tuscan Linguine with rice noodles
- Spaghetti with Marinara Sauce
- Buttered Noodles
- Sautéed Beef
- Braised Beef
- Sautéed Shrimp

Salad

- Chinese Chopped Salad with no wonton strips
- The Mediterranean Salad with no cavatappi noodles
- Cucumber Tomato Salad
- Tossed Green Salad with Balsamic
- Tossed Green Salad with Fat Free Asian

P.F. Changs China Bistro

Please be sure to tell your server that you are ordering off the gluten free menu. Gluten Free options will have a "GF" before the name of the menu option.

Starter

- Chang's chicken lettuce wraps

Salad

- Vietnamese crab salad

Noodles

- Singapore street noodles

Soup

- Egg drop soup

Vegetarian

- Buddha's feast

Rice

- P.F. Chang's fried rice
- Crab fried rice
- P.F. Chang's fried rice combo

Sides

- Spinach stir fried with garlic
- Asian tomato cucumber salad

Entrees

- Shaking beef
- Ginger chicken with broccoli
- Norwegian salmon steamed wit ginger
- Dali chicken
- Chang's spicy chicken
- Moo goo gai pan
- Shrimp with lobster sauce
- Beef a la Sichuan
- Mongolian beef
- Beef with broccoli
- Philips better lemon chicken
- Pepper steak

Dessert

- Flourless chocolate dome

Pei Wei Asian Diner

For the selected menu items below, be sure to order the gluten-free versions.

- Gluten Free Edamame
- Gluten Free Asian Chopped Chicken Salad
- Gluten Free Pei Wei Spicy Chicken Salad
- Gluten Free Pei Wei Spicy Shrimp Salad
- Gluten Free Pei Wei Spicy Salad Combo
- Gluten Free Vietnamese Rolls
- Gluten Free Pei Wei Spicy Chicken
- Gluten Free Pei Wei Spicy Shrimp
- Gluten Free Pei Wei Spicy Combo
- Gluten Free Sweet & Sour Chicken
- Gluten Free Sweet & Sour Shrimp
- Gluten Free Sweet & Sour Combo

Pollo Tropical

Entrée

- Chicken
- Pork
- Shrimp

Sides

- Corn
- Red beans
- Cheddar Cheese

Desserts

- Flan

- Guava Cheesecake

Sauces

- Curry Mustard Sauce

Roy's Hawaiian Fusion

Appetizers

- Roy's original blackened island ahi
- Teppanyaki sesame shrimp
- Crab California roll
- Aloha roll

Greens

- Maui wowie shrimp salad
- Baby greens salad
- Caesar salad

Entrees

- Roasted macadamia nut dusted mahi mahi
- Misoyaki butterfish
- Hibachi grilled salmon
- Blackened island ahi
- Teppanyaki shrimp
- 5 spice hangar steak
- grilled filet mignon
- braised short ribs of beef
- thai style chicken

Tongos

Meats

- Ham
- Turkey
- Salami
- Bacon

Salads

- BBQ Chicken Ranch
- Santa Fe Chicken

Salad Dressings

- Asian
- Balsamic Vinaigrette
- Blue Cheese
- Caesar
- Honey Dijon
- Italian
- Ranch
- Thousand Island

Soups

- Broccoli Cheddar
- Moroccan Lentil

Italian

Just because you can't eat gluten doesn't mean you still can't enjoy a delicious dish of spaghetti and penne meatballs anymore. Thankfully, many Italian restaurants offer the same Italian classics you grew up with, but with a minor gluten free touch.

Bertucci's

Starters

- Vegetable Antipasto
- Grilled Shrimp
- Sausage Soup

Small Plates

- Warm Assorted Olives
- Brick Oven Beets with Blue Cheese
- Roasted Butternut Squash with Candied Walnuts
- Tuscan Roasted Vegetables
- Baked Polenta with Pomodoro without breadcrumbs
- Rosemary Roasted Red Potatoes
- Garlic and Herb Roasted Mushrooms
- Roasted Green Beans

Sharing Salads

You can also add chicken and shrimp to your salads

- Farmhouse Salad
- Roasted Beet and Blue Cheese Salad

Insalata

- Caesar Salad
- Side Insalata
- Side Caesar

Entrées

- Pesto Grilled Salmon
- Cod Al Forno, order without breadcrumbs.
- Filet Mignon with Chianti Sauce

Classic Entrées

- Roasted Eggplant Pomodoro

Dessert

- Chocolate Budino
- Piccolo Chocolate Budino

Biaggi's Ristorante Italiano

Appetizers

- Carpacio
- Mussels in Tomate
- Bacon Wrapped Date

Salads

- House Salad
- Caesar Salad
- Spinach Salad
- Messina Salad
- Roasted Beet Salad

- Chopped Chicken Salad
- Venetian Chicken Salad
- Seared Salmon Salad
- Filet Mignon Salad

Pasta

Brown Rice Gluten Free Pasta (Spaghetti or Penne)

- Pasta Di Mare
- Pasta All Toscana
- Pasta Alfredo
- Pasta Marinara

Pizza

Made with their Gluten Free Dough

- Chicken Picannte
- Sausage Pizza
- Pepperoni Pizza
- Margherita Pizza
- Sicilian Meatball Pizza
- Mediterranean Pizza

Entrées

- Grilled Chicken Parmesan
- Chicken Pietro
- Salmon & Shrimp Milanese
- Potato-Parmesan Crusted Tilapia
- Grilled Pork Chops
- Filet Mignon
- North Atlantic Cod

Gluten Free Sauces

- Alfred

- Bolognese
- Espresso Sauce
- Italian Salsa
- Mac & Cheese Sauce
- Marsala
- Pesto
- Rum Caramel
- Scallion Cream
- Sun-Dried Tomato Cream
- Tomato Sauce

Bravo

Insalata

- Bravo Chopped Salad
- Caesar Salad
- Grilled Salmon Salad

Pasta

- Pasta Pomodoro with Chicken
- Pasta Verduta
- Pasta Bravo

Entrees

- Chicken Griglia
- Grilled Salmon
- Filet Mignon Tosacno

Buca di Beppo

Antipasti and Insalate

- Mussels Bianca or Marinara
- Mozzarella Caprese
- Mixed Green Salad
- Chopped Antipasto Salad
- Apple Gorgonzola Salad
- Di Beppo 1893 Salad

Entrees

- Chicken Limone
- Chicken Saltimbocca
- Veal Saltimbocca
- Salmon Sorrento
- Chicken Marsala
- Veal Marsala

Side Dishes

- Italian Broccoli Romano
- Green Beans
- Rosemary Potatoes
- Sausage and Peppers (mild or spicy)
- Italian Sauce (mild or spicy)

Dessert

- Chocolate ice cream
- Vanilla ice cream

Carrabba's

Below, you'll discover both gluten-free menu items from the Carrabba's gluten free menu, and gluten-free selections from the main menu. Any items with (Gluten Free Menu) means that these items can only be found on the gluten free menu Carrabba's will provide you.

Appetizers

Cozze in Bianco (Gluten Free Menu)

Shrimp Scampi: Request no garlic toast.

Cucina Casuale aka Salads

For all salads, request no croutons and for the salad to be mixed in a fresh bowl.

- Mama Mandola's Sicillian Chicken Soup (Gluten Free Menu): Request no pasta to be added.
- Side Salads: House, Italian, or Caesar
- Carrabba's Caesar Salad: Request the chicken/shrimp to be made without grill baste.
- Italian Cobb Salad: Request the chicken to be made without grill baste.

Marsala (Gluten Free Menu)

Be sure to request that the marsala to be made without grill baste. Served with a cup of homemade soup or a side salad.

- Chicken
- Sirloin
- Pork Chop

Classics & Combinations

Served with a cup of homemade soup or a side salad. Request to be made without grill baste.

- The Johnny
- Chicken Trio

Wood-Burning Grill

Served with a cup of homemade soup or a side salad. Request to be made without grill baste.

- Chicken Bryan (Gluten Free Menu)
- Grilled Salmon
- Pollo Rosa Maria (Gluten Free Menu)
- Grilled Chicken
- Filet Fiorentina

Dessert

- John Cole

The Old Spaghetti Factory

Be sure to request gluten-free pasta. There is a small additional charge for the gluten-free pasta however.

Starters

- Salad

Pasta Classics

Choose one or a combination of the following sauces with the gluten free pasta.

- Marinara
- Riche Mea
- Clam
- Alfredo
- Sautéed Mushroom
- Mizithra Cheese & Browned Butter and Marinara Sauce

Just For Kids

Choose one of the following sauces with the gluten free pasta:

- Macaroni & Cheese Style Sauce
- Marinara
- Riche Mea
- Clam
- Sautéed Mushroom
- Mizithra Cheese & Browned Butter and Marinara Sauce

Side Orders

- Whole seasoned all natural chicken breast
- Italian sausage
- Marinated diced all natural chicken

Beverages

- Italian Cream Soda

Desserts

- Ice Cream: Vanilla or Spumoni

Olive Garden

Please be sure to ask your server for the Gluten-Free version of their menu.

Salads

- Garden Fresh Salad: Order without croutons
- Caesar Salad: Order without croutons

Pastas

Be sure to request Gluten-Free Pasta

- Penne Rigate Pomodoro
- Penne Rigate with Marinara
- Children's Penne Rigate with Marinara

Entrees

- Steak Toscano
- Herb-Grilled Salmon
- Mixed Grill
- Mixed Grill (Chicken)
- Children's Grilled Chicken

Sides and Garnishes

- Broccoli
- Side of Grapes
- Grilled Vegetables
- Red Bell Peppers

Romano's Macaroni Grill

For all pasta dishes, be sure to request the gluten-free penne.

Tapas & Antipasti aka Appetizers

- Baked Prosciutto & Mozzarella
- Chianti Sausage & Crispy Potatoes
- Mediterranean Olives

Soups

- Clam Chowder: Order without Pasta Chips
- Lentil Soup
- Minestrone Soup without pasta
- Pormodorina Soup without Crostini

Pantry aka Salads

- Bibb & Blue without crispy onions
- Caesar without croutons
- Caprese
- Fresh Greens without croutons
- Market Chop without breadstick
- Warm Spinach & Shrimp

Salad Dressings

- Balsamic Vinaigrette
- Caesar
- Mediterranean Vinaigrette
- Parmesan Peppercorn Ranch

Pasta

Be sure to order the Gluten-Free Penne Pasta

- Carbonara

- Carmela's Chicken
- Pasta di Mare
- Pasta Milano
- Penne Rustica
- Shrimp Portofino

Italian Classics

- Fettuccine Alfredo: Order with Gluten-Free Penne Pasta

Pollo aka Chicken

- Chicken Under a Brick without potatoes
- Grilled Chicken Spiedini without vegetables
- Pollo Caprese with Gluten-Free Penne Pasta

Pesce aka Fish

- Grilled King Salmon: Order without orzo
- Grilled Shrimp Spiedini without vegetables

Carne aka Meat

- Pan-Roasted Pork Chop: Order without risotto

Kids Menu

- Fettuccine Alfredo: Order with Gluten-Free Penne Pasta
- Grilled Chicken & Pasta: Order with Gluten-Free Penne Pasta
- Mac & Cheese: Order with Gluten-Free Penne Pasta
- Spaghetti & Pomodor: Order with Gluten-Free Penne Pasta

Sides

- Bibb & Blue: Order without crispy onions
- Caesar Salad: Order without croutons
- Fresh Greens Salad: Order without croutons

- Grilled Asparagus
- Spinach & Garlic

Create Your Own Pasta

Be sure to order with the Gluten-Free Penne Pasta

Sauces

- Alfredo
- Arrabbiata Sauce
- Garlic Cream Sauce/Garlic Olive Oil
- Promodoro Sauce

Top It Off

- Artichokes
- Asparagus
- Broccolini
- Cannellini Beans
- Caramelized Onions
- Fresh Spinach
- Roasted Garlic
- Roasted Mushrooms
- Roasted Peppers
- Roasted Tomatoes
- Snap Peas
- Sun-Dried Tomatoes

Add

- Italian Sausage
- Pancetta
- Roasted Chicken
- Shrimp

Dolce aka Desserts

- Dark Chocolate Gelato without biscotti
- Double Vanilla Gelato without biscotti
- Sorbet

Mexican, Hispanic, & Southwest

If you're a sucker for tacos, enchiladas, burritos, Mexican rice and beans, and the classic chips & salsa, you'll find everything you can think of in this section.

Abuelo's Mexican Food Embassy

Be sure to request a special gluten-free menu.

Starters & Salads

- Guacamole Salad
- Garden Salad
- Shrimp Fajita Salad

Tex-Mex

- Soft Taco Plate
- Tamale Plate

House Specialties

- Ribeye Steak
- Pork Tenderloin with Honey Chile Glaze
- Alambre de Camaron
- Salmon Santa Cruz

Fajitas

- Bacon-Wrapped Stuffed Shrimp
- Pork Tenderloin
- Vegetarian
- Pescado

Dessert

- Traditional Flan

Austin Grill

Appetizers

- Austin Wings
- Michoacan Tamales Plate
- Homemade Guacamole
- Longhorn Nachos

Entrees

- Grilled Salmon Salad
- Cheese Enchiladas
- Migas Plate
- Carne Asada Steak
- Carnita Fajitas
- Huevos Rancheros
- Grille Vegetable Enchiladas

Baja Fresh

- Baja Tacos made with corn tortillas
- Any "Bare style" burrito
- Baja Ensalada with choice of steak, chicken, or grilled shrimp, as well as grilled vegetables, carnitas, rice, and both varieties of beans
- All dressings
- All salsas

Blue Mesa Grill

Starters/Appetizers

- Tableside Guacamole
- Texas Toothpicks with Queso (no chicken, shrimp or Mesa Panna Bread; salmon has a cornmeal crust*)
- Queso Blanco

Salads

- Avocado, Mango & Jicama Salad with Grilled Shrimp
- Southwestern Caesar – (plain or salmon only, no croutons)

Entrees

- Adobe Pie (both chicken and black bean-cheese are made with corn*)
- Southwestern Fajitas (steak only, no tortillas)
- Mixed Grill Churrascaritas (steak and sausage only, no Mesa Panna Bread)
- Blue Mesa Churrascaritas (steak only, no Mesa Panna Bread)
- Spa Churrascaritas (steak only)
- Free Range Chicken with Roasted Serrano Pesto (seasonal vegetable varies)
- Carne Asada (seasonal vegetable varies)

Seafood

- Spa Grilled Fish-of-the-Day
- Red Chile Crusted Salmon (has a cornmeal crust*)
- Baja Shrimp (seasonal vegetable varies)

Veggies

- Vegetable Sampler (seasonal vegetable varies)

- Sweet Potato-Black Bean-Goat Cheese Chile Relleno with a veggie skewer (a la carte)

Sauces

- Three Chile Sauce
- Chipotle Cream
- Tomatillo Sauce
- Avocado Sauce
- Red Table Salsa
- Fire Roasted Salsa

Dessert

- Tres Flans (ask about changing flavors)

Café Rio

Entrees

- Nachos with Grilled Meat and no beans
- Salad without Tortilla, rice and beans, with Grilled Meat
- Tostada with Grilled Meat and no rice and beans

Sauces and Sides

- Pico
- Fresca
- Guacamole

Dessert

- Coconut or Chocolate Flan

Chevys Fresh Mex

Appetizers

- Guacamole
- Chips: Please call in advance so they can fry in separate oil to prevent cross-contamination

Salsa

- Chile Con Queso Dip
- Chicken Tamale
- Tableside Guacamole

Appetizer Accompaniments

- Jalapeño jelly
- Pineapple salsa
- Sour cream
- Pico de gallo

Fresh Salads

- Sante Fe Chopped Salad without tortilla strips, bacon or marinade on chicken
- Fajita Grilled Chicken Salad without tortilla strips, bacon, or marinade on the chicken

Salad Dressings

- Salsa vinaigrette
- Ranch
- Chipotle Apple Vinaigrette

Fajitas

- Succulent Shrimp: Corn tortillas only
- Chicken Fajitas without marinade

- Fresh Catch of the Day without marinade

Fajita Accompaniments

- Guacamole
- Sour cream
- Pico de gallo
- Rice
- Beans (black, charra/pinto)
- Sweet corn tamalito
- Corn tortillas

Fresh Mex Specialties

- Order with corn tortillas
- Chicken Tacos
- Steak Tacos
- Beef Taco
- Chicken Taco
- Chicken Tamale

Sauces

- Ranchero Sauce
- Green Sauce
- Kiddie Meals
- Beef or Chicken Taco: Request unfried corn tortilla
- Kiddie Cheeseburger: No bun

Desserts

- Chevys Flan with no cactus garnish
- Chiquita Sundae: No tortilla shell; no cactus garnish
- Kiddie Kone: Ice cream only

Chipotle

Meats and Taco Shell

- Barbacoa
- Chicken
- Camitas
- Steak
- Crispy Taco Shell

Toppings

- Cilantro Lime Rice
- Black Beans
- Pinto Beans
- Fajita Vegetables
- Tomato Salsa
- Corn Salsa
- Red Tomatillo Salso
- Cheese
- Sour Cream
- Guacamole
- Romaine Lettuce
- Chips
- Vinaigrette
- Soft Corn Tortilla
- Breakfast Eggs
- Breakfast Relish
- Breakfast Chorizo
- Breakfast Potatoes

Del Taco

Entree

- Plain hamburger patty

Sauces

- CRed Sauce
- Green Sauce

Sides, Toppings, and Shells

- Taco Shells
- Tortilla Shells
- Lettuce
- Tomato
- Onion
- Cheddar cheese
- Spicy Jack Cheese

Dessert

- Vanilla Shake

Don Pablos

Please be sure to alert the manager of your allergy prior to placing an order.

Dips

Available with corn tortillas

- Prairie Fire Bean Dip: Order without flour tortilla
- Queso Dip

- Table Salsa

Fresh Salads

Available with table salsa or red wine vinegar and soy salad oil

- Sizzling Fajita Salad
- Taco Salad: Request no crisp flour tortilla bowl
- Red River Salad: Request no honey lime dressing with gilled steak instead of chicken.
- Tortilla Salad: Request no crisp flour tortilla bowl

Classic Fajitas

Request corn tortillas

- Grilled Shrimp
- Grilled Steak
- Shrimp & Steak
- Pecos Valley Veggie
- Portabella Mushroom: Request no chipotle butter

Don's Combos

"Skinny Style"- corn tortillas that are softened in water versus fryer oil

- Cinco Combo: Request crispy instead of soft chicken taco, red sauce instead of chili meat sauce on beef enchilada and "skinny style" enchiladas
- Mexicano: Request red sauce instead of chili meat sauce on beef enchilada and "skinny style" enchiladas
- Tejas: Request "skinny style" enchiladas

Create Your Own Combos

Request red sauce instead of chili meat sauce on beef enchilada and "skinny style" for all enchiladas

- Crispy Tacos: Beef or Chicken
- Enchilada: Mama's Skinny, Cheese, Chicken, or Beef

Kids' Menu

- Crispy Tacos: Beef or Chicken
- Steak Fajitas: Request corn tortillas
- Cheese Enchilada: Request "skinny style" enchilada

Tastes of Mexico

Request "skinny style" corn tortillas

- Big Tex Ribeye
- Grilled Tilapia
- Grilled Shrimp: Request sour cream sauce on shrimp instead of cilantro-lime or Diablo sauce
- Carnitas: Request corn instead of flour tortillas
- Steak & Enchiladas: Request "skinny style" enchiladas

Gluten Free Sauces

- Ranchero
- Santa Fe Red Chile
- Regular Salsa
- Sour Cream
- Cholula

Gluten Free Sides

- Mexican Rice
- Seasoned Vegetables
- Chile Mashed Potatoes
- Charra Beans
- Refritos
- Prairie Fire Beans

Beverages

- SqueezeRita
- PabloRita
- LotsaRita
- PrimaRita

El Pollo Loco

Meats

- Flame grilled Mexican chicken
- Corn Tortillas

Sides and Toppings

- Pinto Beans
- Refried beans
- Avocado Salsa
- Cotija Cheese
- Mixed Vegetables

Dessert

- Flan

Jimboys

Anything with Flour Tortillas, Burger Buns, or our Enchilada Sauce most likely contains Gluten. The above list is only what we know for certain is free of it. Food is NOT cooked in a gluten free environment.

Tacos

- Bean

- Ground Beef
- Chicken
- Steak
- Carnitas

Tacoburger

- Taquitos
- Ground Beef
- Chicken

Tostadas

- Bean
- Ground Beef
- Chicken
- Steak

Kid's Menu

- Ground Beef Taco

Quick Snacks

- Ground Beef Pepper Poppers

The Works

- Guacamole & Sour Cream

Mighty Taco

Tacos

Use the Corn Shell only.

- Mighty Taco with Seasoned Ground Beef
- Mighty Taco with Seasoned Ground Chicken
- Mighty Pack with Seasoned Ground Chicken
- Seasoned Ground Beef and Cheese
- Seasoned Ground Chicken and Cheese
- Seasoned Ground Beef, Refried Bean and Cheese
- Seasoned Ground Chicken, Refried Bean and Cheese
- Refried Bean and Cheese
- Meatless Mighty
- Veggies and Cheese

Extras

- Lettuce
- Tomato
- Banana Peppers
- Nacho Cheese
- Cheddar Cheese
- Swiss and American Cheese
- Guacamole
- Salsa
- Sour Cream
- Peppers and Onions
- Crumbled Tortilla Chips
- Refried Beans
- Seasoned Ground Chicken
- Seasoned Ground Beef
- Fajita Chicken
- Buffito Chicken

Salads

- Taco Beef Salad
- Mighty Chicken Salad
- Chicken Fajita Salad
- Chicken Buffito Salad

Salad Dressing

- Ranch
- Blue Cheese
- Italian
- Raspberry Vinaigrette

Sides

- Bean Dip
- Nachos Deluxe with Seasoned Ground Beef
- Nachos Deluxe with Seasoned Ground Chicken
- Refried Beans
- Strip Chips
- Strip Chips and Guacamole
- Strip Chips and Salsa
- Strip Chips and Nacho Cheese

Certified Gluten Free Products

- Buffito Chicken
- Fajita Chicken
- Swiss American Cheese
- Sharp Cheddar Cheese
- Sour Cream
- Guacamole
- Strip Chips
- Ken's: Ranch, Blue Cheese, Italian, Raspberry Vinaigrette Dressing

Moe's Southwest Grill

Meats and Proteins

- Chicken
- Steak
- Ground Beef
- Pork
- Tofu
- Fish

Beans

- Black beans
- Pinto Beans

Toppings and Extras

- Black olives
- Cheese
- Chipotle ranch
- Cucumbers
- Guacamole
- Jalapenos
- Lettuce
- Cheese (Queso)
- Rice
- Salsa (Kaiser and El Guapo)
- Sour Cream
- Southwest Vinaigrette
- Veggies
- Tomatillo Salsa
- Pico de Gallo
- Corn Pico de Gallo
- Hard Rock 'N Roll Sauce

On the Border Mexican Grill & Cantina

Appetizers

- Served without Tortilla Strips
- Con Queso: Chile, Carne Style
- Guacamole & Guacamole Live

Salads

Listed without Dressing and Tortilla Strips

- Citrus Chipotle Chicken
- House Salad
- Sizzling Fajita Salad: Chicken or Steak without Sour Cream and Onions.

Salad Dressings

- Chipotle Honey Mustard
- Fat Free Mango Citrus Vinaigrette
- Ranch
- Smoked Jalapeño Vinaigrette

Fajita Grill

All listed without condiments, onions, and flour tortillas

- Fajitas
- Mesquite Grilled Chicken
- Mesquite Grilled Steak
- Pork Carnita

Sauces

- Chile Con Queso
- Red-Chile-Tomatillo Salsa
- Fresh Grill

- Chicken Salsa Fresca
- Jalapeño BBQ Salmon
- Queso Chicken
- Tomatillo Chicken

Tacos

All listed without any sides

- Achiote Chicken
- Grilled Fish
- Street-Style (Mini): Chicken or Steak

Sides and Extras

- Black Beans
- Black Bean & Corn Salsa
- Cilantro Lime Rice
- Corn Tortilla
- Grilled Vegetables
- Guacamole
- Mexican Rice
- Mixed Cheese
- Pico
- Refried Beans without Blue Corn Chips
- Sautéed Vegetables
- Sour Cream

Sauces

- Chile Con Queso
- Green Chile
- Jalapeño BBQ
- Salsa

Kids Menu

All listed without any sides

- Kids Grilled Chicken Entrée
- Kids House Salad without Dressing (Choose form one of the gluten-free dressings as seen above)
- Kids Mixed Vegetables
- Kids Dessert: Chocolate or Strawberry Sundae

Beverages

- Borderita Grande
- Fresh Lime Skinny Margarita
- Grande Herradura Margarita
- House Margarita
- Mexican Martini
- Mojito
- Perfect Patron
- Red and White Wine
- Sangria
- Sangria Swirl Margarita
- Shaken Margarita
- Strawberry Lemonade

Qdoba

Entrée

- Soft White Corn Tortilla
- Cilantro Lime Rice
- Black Beans
- Pork
- Chicken
- Ground Sirloin
- Seasoned Shredded Beef
- Flat Iron Steak
- Chorizo
- Eggs

- Tortilla Soup

Salsas and Dressings

- Poblano Pesto
- 3 Cheese Queso
- Ranchera
- Guacamole
- Lite Sour Cream
- Fat Free Ranch Dressing
- Fat Free Picante Ranch Dressing
- Cilantro Lime Vinaigrette

Rubio's

Entrees

- Grilled or Blackened Atlantic Salmon Taco
- Grilled or Blackened Pacific Mahi Mahi Taco
- Grilled Gourmet Taco with Shrimp
- Grilled Gourmet Taco with Steak
- Classic Grilled Steak Taco
- Grilled or Blackened Regal Springs Tilapia Taco
- Grilled Grande Bow with Shrimp
- Chipotle Orange Bowl
- Salsa Verde Shrimp Taco with Corn Tortilla
- Rubio's Street Tacos with Steak

Salads

For all the salads, substitute the grilled chicken with shrimp, grilled or blackened salmon, mahi mahi, or tilapia. Or request with no chicken.

- Balsamic and Roasted Veggie Salad
- Chopped Salad

- Chipotle Ranch Salad
- Grilled Grande Bowl

Sides

- Chips
- Applesauce
- Bacon
- Black Beans
- Chicken Tortilla Soup Broth
- Guacamole
- Jalapeños
- Mexican Rice
- Pinto Beans
- Serrano Slaw
- Sour Cream
- Spring Mix

Dressings, Salsas, and Sauces

- Balsamic Vinaigrette Dressing
- Chipotle Orange Dressing
- Chipotle Ranch Dressing
- Crena
- Creamy Chipotle Sauce
- Fire Roasted Corn
- Mango Pineapple Salsa
- Mild Salsa
- Picante Salsa
- Red Chile Sauce
- Roasted Chipotle Salsa
- Salsa Fresca
- Salsa Verde
- Tomatillo Salsa
- White Sauce

Taco Bell

- Pintos 'n Cheese
- Mexican Rice
- Tostada

Taco John's

Due to shared fryers and a high risk of cross contamination, this is not a safe place for anyone on a medical gluten free diet.

Entrees

- Crispy Taco
- Crispy Taco with Cheese
- Super Nachos

Sides

- Nachos
- Chili without Crackers
- Chili without Crackers and Cheese
- Refried Beans

Sauces and Condiments

- Mild Sauce
- Hot Sauce
- Super Hot Sauce
- Pico de Gallo
- Salsa
- Sour Cream X
- Guacamole
- Nacho Cheese Sauce
- House Dressing

- Ranch Dressing
- Bacon Ranch Dressing
- Creamy Italian Dressing

Taco Time

Entrée

With the corn tortilla taco shell, please understand that these are fried in the same fryers as other non-gluten free foods so there is a large risk of cross contamination. You can however ask for your corn tortilla to be warmed up using the microwave.

- Crispy Ground Beef Taco with or without sour cream
- Ground Beef Enchilada

Sides

- Chips
- Cheddar Fries
- Mexi-Fries
- Mexi-Rice
- Refritos with Chips

Sauces and Dressings

- Sour Cream
- Guacamole
- Salsa Fresca
- Salsa Nuevo
- Salsa Verde
- Chipotle Ranch Dressing
- Ranch Dressing
- Thousand Island Dressing

Pizza

No, this isn't a typo. Pizza is back on the menu! Just because you can't eat gluten doesn't mean you can't enjoy a fresh slice of thin crust pizza. With a majority of pizza joints starting to add a gluten free pizza to their menu, you can now enjoy that pepperoni pizza you've been craving for months.

California Pizza Kitchen

Gluten Free Pizza

- Original Barbecue Chicken
- Pepperoni
- Mushroom Pepperoni Sausage
- Margherita

Small Plates + Appetizers

- Asparagus + Arugula Salad
- White Corn Guacamole + Chips
- Petite Wedge

Salads

- Caramelized Peach
- Roasted Veggie
- Italian Chopped
- California Cobb
- Moroccan-Spiced Chicken
- Waldorf Chicken
- Field Greens

CPKIDS aka Kids Menu

- Fresh fruit
- Kids Sundae

Domino's

Although the gluten free crust on the Domino's gluten free menu, is gluten free, it's made in-house meaning that it's basically made in the same kitchen, on the same table, as the rest of the glutenous pizzas and toppings.

So if you're just on a gluten free diet and don't really worry about cross-contamination, then the Domino's gluten free crust should be a good option for any of you in the mood for pizza.

Crust

Be sure to get the Domino's gluten free pizza crust.

- Domino's gluten free crust

Sauces

- BBQ
- Hearty Marinara
- Hot Sauce
- Mango Habanero
- Ranch Dressing
- Robust Inspired Tomato Sauce
- White Sauce

Meat

- Bacon
- Beef

- Ham
- Italian Sausage
- Pepperoni
- Premium Chicken
- Salami
- Sliced Italian Sausage

Other Toppings

- American Cheese
- Banana Peppers
- Black Olives
- Cheddar Cheese
- Cheese
- Diced Tomatoes
- Feta Cheese
- Green Peppers
- Hot Sauce
- Jalapenos
- Mushroom
- Onions
- Pineapples
- Roasted Red Peppers
- Shredded Parmesan Asiago
- Shredded Provolone Cheese
- Sliced Provolone Cheese
- Spinach

Donatos

Donatos features Gluten Free Pizza using Udi's Gluten Free Crust.

Signature Pizza Combinations

- Pepperoni

- Serious Cheese
- Classic Trio
- Hawaiian
- Mariachi
- Chicken
- Mariachi Beef
- Vegy
- The Works
- Serious Meat

Founder's Favorite

- Fresh Mozzarella Trio
- Margherita
- Chicken Spinach
- Mozzarella
- Pepperoni Zinger

Create Your Own Topping Choices

Sauce

- Olive oil
- Thin sauce
- Thick sauce

Protein

- Pepperoni
- Ham
- Bacon
- Family Recipe Sausage
- Beef
- Chicken

Cheese

- Aged Smoked Provolone

- Cheddar
- Three Cheese Blend
- Romano Parmesan Blend
- Fresh Mozzarella
- Bleu Cheese Crumbles

Pizza Toppings

- Onion
- Green Pepper
- Spinach
- Roma Tomato
- Mushrooms
- Green/Black Olive
- Garlic
- Jalapeño
- Pineapple
- Basil

Traditional Bone-In Wings

- Hot
- Mild
- BBQ
- Garlic

Salads

- Italian Chef Side and Entrée

Salad Dressings

- Italian
- Buttermilk Ranch
- Fat Free
- Ranch
- Apple Vinaigrette
- Lt. Italian

- Honey French
- Bleu Cheese

Extreme Pizza

Be sure to order the gluten free pizza crust.

Signature Pizzas

- Green with Envy
- The Screamin Tomato
- Baja 1000
- White Out
- Mr Pestato Head
- Railroad Grade
- Peace in the Middle East
- Pandora's Box
- Drag it Thru the Garden
- Ragin Rooster
- The Boar'der
- Yard Sale
- Paia Pie

Gluten Free Fresh Salads

- Spinach Salad
- Fresh Tracks
- Greek Salad
- Back Country Betty

6666666

Figaro's Pizza

Crust

- Gluten Free Crust

Sauce

- Original Red

Toppings

- Salami
- Pepperoni
- Sausage
- Beef
- Chicken
- Pineapples
- Mushrooms
- Black Olives
- Onions
- Jalapenos
- Tomatoes
- Green Peppers
- 100% Real Cheese

Garlic Jim's

Be sure to order the gluten free crust!

Specialty Pizzas

- Garlic Jims Ultimate
- Nutty Chipotle
- Jim's Smokin Sweet BBQ Chicken
- Gourmet Hawaiian

- The Hercules
- Southwestern Chicken
- Queen Margherita
- Spinach Artichoke Pie
- Jim's Veggies
- Chicken Bacon Ranch

Build Your Own Pizza

- *Cheeses*: fresh whole milk mozzarella, cheddar, feta, grated parmesan
- *Sauces*: classic red, smokin sweet BBQ, basil pesto, zesty chipotle pesto, olive oil, creamy ranch
- *Meats*: pepperoni, spicy italian sausage, canadian bacon, grilled chicken, salami, beef, bacon, anchovies
- *Vegetables*: green peppers, red onions, pineapple, roma tomatoes, mushrooms, black olives, jalapenos
- *Gourmet Toppings*: Roasted garlic, marinated artichoke hearts, roasted corn, fresh basil, spinach, black beans, sun dried tomatoes, coconut, almond slivers, cashews.

Gourmet Extras

- House Salad
- Chop Salad
- Southwest Chipotle Chicken Salad
- Hot Wings (don't get BBQ wings, contains gluten)
- Ribs
- Jim's Gourmet Cheesecake (and yes, it's gluten free)
- Gourmet Ice Cream

Godfather's Pizza

Be sure to order the gluten-free dough/crust.

Toppings

- Cheese
- Pepperoni
- Sausage
- All-Meat Combo
- Beef
- Classic Combo

Mellow Mushroom

Be sure to order the 12" gluten free pizza crust.

Specialty Pies aka Pizza

- House Special
- Gourmet White
- Mighty Meaty
- Veg Out
- Kosmic Karma
- Cheese Pizza

Build Your Own/Add Your Favorite Gluten-Free Ingredients

- *Bases/Sauces*: Red Sauce, Olive Oil, Olive Garlic, Garlic, Pest
- *Veggies*: black olives, green peppers, button mushrooms, onions, spinach, sun-dried tomatoes, fresh tomatoes
- *Cheeses*: mozzarella, feta, provolone, vegan cheese (daiya)

- *Proteins*: bacon, ground beef, ham, Italian sausage, pepperoni

Picazzo

The best thing about Picazzo is that almost everything on the menu has a gluten free alternative.

Gluten Free Appetizers

- Artisan Bruschetta
- Classic stuffed peppers with spicy sausage
- Three mama's meat-za balls
- Caprese
- Baked brie and roasted garlic
- Hot artichoke spinach dip
- Baked Portobello mushroom cap
- Five baked artichoke bottoms
- Organic garlic cheese bread
- Organic hummus platter
- Baked wings: buffalo, oven-roasted, BBQ chipotle, BBQ maple, Super Hot Chipotle, Spicy Thai Peanut Sauce

Gluten Free Organic Salads

- *Proteins*: chicken, pancetta, ham, Italian chopped meat mix, shrimp
- *Fruits and vegetables*: avocado figs, dates, grilled Portobello
- Heart healthy gourmet
- Chopped kale
- Kaie Caesar
- Organic Caesar
- Award winning Greek
- Berry-licious

- Fresh pear gogonzola
- Natural chopped Italian
- Picazzo's organic wedge
- Bleu cheese
- Spinach
- Mixed green salad
- The Asian

Organic and Gluten Free Pasta

- Seven veggie pasta
- Avocado delish
- Wild mushroom rotelli
- Chicken picatta
- Spaghetti and meatballs
- Uncle louie's favorite
- Pasta Bianca
- Spicy thai peanut chicken
- Spicy indian curry chicken
- Chipotle chicken
- Rotelli pesto and chicken
- Shrimp scampi

Baked Organic and Gluten Free Dishes and Ravioli

- Lasagna Bolognese
- Vegetable lasagna
- Eggplant parmesan
- Three baked cannelloni
- Three baked spinach ricotta cannelloni
- Five cheese ravioli
- Butternut squash ravioli
- Pesto and ravioli
- Ravioli carbonara
- Ravioli with fresh vegetables

Neopolitan Pizzas (12" only)

- Fig gorgonzola
- Pancetta and caramelized onions
- Chicken indian curry
- Artichoke bottoms and hearts
- Sweet and sassy
- Rock shrimp
- Fresh mozzarella and cherry tomato
- Wild mushroom and spinach
- Milano
- California
- Naples margherita

Specialty Gourmet Pizzas

Be sure to order a medium gluten free pizza.

- Tarragon chicken
- Roasted Anaheim pepper and chicken
- BBQ chicken
- Chipotle and chicken
- Thai chicken
- Free range chicken pesto
- Double pepperoni
- Meaty meaty
- The vortex
- Hawaiian
- Pepperoni, sausage and ricotta
- Pesto classic
- Diavola
- Awesome avocado
- Super veggie
- Margherita
- Vegetarian
- Puttanesca
- Nonna's favorite

Gluten Free Side Dishes

- Veggies
- Tender broccoli crowns
- Sautéed spinach
- Marinated mixed veggies
- Fresh berry bowl

Pizza Fusion

Pizza Crust

- House-made Gluten Free Pizza Crust

Toppings

- All toppings except sausage

Sauces

- All sauces except barbecue sauce

Salad

- All salads without croutons

Dessert

- Gluten free brownie

Pizza Pie Café

Pizza

- Gluten-free pizza crust

Sauce

- Pizza sauce
- Marinara sauce
- BBQ sauce
- Basil Pesto

Pizza Toppings

- Pepperoni
- Canadian bacon
- Crisp bacon
- Thick potato slices
- Fresh mushrooms
- Dole pineapples
- Black olives
- Green peppers
- Sweet red onions
- Fresh roma tomatoes
- Chives
- Jalapeños
- Chipotle seasoning

Salad

All salad toppings are gluten free EXCEPT:

- Croutons
- Bacon bits
- Sunflower seeds
- Goldfish
- Dressings
- Italian dressing
- Thousand Island dressing
- Blue cheese

Pasta

- Request gluten-free pasta at the pasta bar

Pasta Sauces

- Marinara
- Meat marinara

Sam & Louie's New York Pizzeria

Salads

All dressings are gluten-free. Order without croutons.

- Sam's Cobb Salad
- Original Chicken Salad
- Chicken Caesar
- Sam's House Salad
- Side Caesar

Pizza

Be sure to get the gluten free pizza dough.

- Sam and Louie's Best
- Buffalo Jack
- Veggie
- Five Cheese
- Carnivore
- Combo
- BBQ Chicken
- Fire Ball
- Chicken Bacon Ranch
- Bacon Cheeseburger
- California Pie

- Hawaiian Luau
- Brooklyn

Create Your Own Pizza

Be sure to request gluten-free dough

Cheeses

- Ricotta
- Feta
- Romano
- Bleu cheese crumbles
- Cheddar
- Extra cheese

Fruits and Vegetables

- Broccoli
- Black olive
- Green olive
- Green bell pepper
- Red bell pepper
- Jalapeño
- Pineapple
- Red onion
- Mushroom
- Sliced roma tomatoes
- Garlic
- Spinach

Meats

- Italian sausage
- Buffalo chicken
- Grilled chicken
- Canadian bacon
- Pepperoni

- Salami
- Bacon
- Beef

Uno's Chicago Grill

Steak and Seafood

- Top Sirloin Steak
- New York Strip Steak
- Salmon with Chimichurri
- Lemon Basil Salmon
- Grilled Shrimp and Sirloin

Pizza

- Cheese
- Pepperoni
- Veggie
- Chicken
- Herb-Rubbed Breast of Chicken
- Baked Stuffed Spinoccoli

Soup

- Chili
- Cuban Black Bean and Lentil

Salads

- Garden Salad
- Classic Cobb Salad
- Caesar Salad
- Chicken Caesar Salad

Dressings

- Caesar
- Ranch
- Classic Vinaigrette
- Fat-Free Vinaigrette
- Honey Mustard
- Bleu Cheese
- Balsamic Vinaigrette
- Low Fat Pomegranate Vinaigrette
- Honey-Lime

Burgers

- The Uno Burger on an Udi's Gluten Free Roll
- Guac-alicious Burger on an Udi's Gluten Free Roll

Sides

- Whole grain brown rice
- Red bliss mashed potatoes
- Steamed broccoli
- Roasted seasonal vegetables
- Skinless baked

Freezers

- Strawberry Smoothie
- Chocolate Monkey
- Tropical Fruity Freezer
- Raspberry Lime Ricky
- Wildberry Mango Smoothie

Desserts

- Ice Cream Sundae
- Beer
- Brunehaut

- Woodchuck cider

Your Pie

Dough

- Gluten Free

Sauce

- BBQ
- Basil Pesto
- Garlic Olive Oil
- Hot
- Marinara
- Ranchy Marinara
- Sundried Tomato
- Thai

Cheese

- Cheddar
- Feta
- Fresh Mozzarella (Circles)
- Gorgonzola
- Low Fat Mozzarella
- Mozzarella
- Parmesan
- Provolone
- Ricotta
- Vegan Cheese

Premium Ingredients

- Anchovies
- Artichoke Hearts

- Bacon
- Capicola
- Chicken
- Dried Cranberries
- Ham
- Pecans
- Pepperoni
- Roasted Red Peppers
- Salami
- Sundried Tomato
- Tofu
- Turkey

Fresh Ingredients

- Banana Peppers
- Basil
- Black Olives
- Broccoli
- Carrots
- Cilantro
- Corn
- Roasted Garlic
- Green Olives
- Green Peppers
- Jalapeños
- Baby Bellas (Mushrooms)
- Oregano
- Pineapple
- Red Onions
- Romaine
- Spinach
- Tomatoes
- Vidalia Onions (White)

zpizza

Pizza Crust

- Gluten-free crust

Cheese

- Mozzarella cheese
- Vegan cheese
- Feta cheese

Sauce

- Organic Tomato sauce
- Marinara sauce
- Chipotle pesto
- Basil pesto
- BBQ sauce
- Mango Chutney
- Roasted garlic sauce
- Mexican salsa

Vegetables

- All fresh vegetables
- Greek olive mix

Meats

- Pepperoni
- Italian Sausage
- Salamis
- All-natural chicken breast
- BBQ Chicken
- Lime chicken

Dressings

- Girard's Caesar dressing
- Girard's Old Venice Italian
- Girard's Balsamic
- Girard's Ranch

Pub Style, Grill, & Barbecue

BBQ joints, sport grills, and breweries, oh my! Some of the most popular chain restaurants in the U.S. can be found in this section.

Applebee's

Appetizers

- Chips & Salsa
- Queso Blanco

Steaks

- New York Strip
- Ribeye

Steak Toppers

- Grilled Onions

Soup

- Tuscan Bean Soup with Chicken & Sausage

Sides

- Baked Potato (Regular and Loaded)
- French Fries
- Signature Cole Slaw
- Fruit Side
- Garlic Mashed Potatoes (Regular and Loaded)
- Seasonal Vegetables
- Almond Rice Pilaf
- Mexi Rice

- Celery
- Applesauce
- Herb Potatoes
- Add Grilled Shrimp
- Crispy Red Potatoes

Chicken

- Napa Chicken & Portobellos
- Fiesta Lim Chicken
- Bourbon Street Chicken & Shrimp

Salads

- Grilled Shrimp 'N Spinach Salad
- Fiesta Chicken Chopped Salad

Salad Dressings

- Ranch
- Creamy Bleu Cheese
- Fat-Free Italian
- Garlic Caesar Dressing
- Honey Balsamic
- Honey French
- Honey Mustard
- Mexi Ranch
- Oriental Vinaigrette
- Jalapeño Dressing
- Champagne Vinaigrette

Seafood

- Blackened Tilapia
- Grilled Jalapeño-Lime Shrimp
- Sizzling N'Awlins Skillet

Sauces

- Pico de Gallo
- Southern Barbecue
- Guacamole
- Marinara
- Salsa
- Bruschetta
- Balsamic Glaze
- Black Bean Corn Salsa
- Mayonnaise
- Sour Cream
- Napa Valley Red Wine Sauce
- Chunky Roma Pepper Relish
- Pesto Mayo
- Chimichurri Sauce
- Alfredo Sauce
- Honey Barbecue Sauces

BJ's Restaurant and Brewhouse

Garden Fresh Specialty Salads

- Santa Fe Salad without tortilla strips
- Garden Medley Salad: Also available with grilled chicken or blackened salmon
- Italian Market Salad
- House Wedge Salad
- House Salad: No croutons
- House Caesar Salad without croutons
- BBQ Chicken Chopped Salad without onion strings

Gluten-Free Thin Crust Pizza

- A flavorful, herb infused, 10-inch crust baked to a golden brown and topped with your favorite gluten-free toppings. All BJ's Classic Ingredients are gluten free, except for meatballs.

Soup

- Tuscan Tomato Bisque without croutons
- Broccoli Cheddar

Giant Stuffed Potatoes

- Garden Vegetable Potato without Alfredo sauce
- Grilled Chicken Potato without Alfredo cheese
- The "Classic" Baked Potato

Specialty Entrees

- Flame-Broiled New York Strip
- Fresh Atlantic Salmon without Chardonnay butter sauce and rice pilaf.

Weekend Brunch

- BJ's California Scramble: No toast and country potatoes.

Culinary Creations

- Balsamic Glazed Chicken: No onion strings.

Breakfast Sides

- Country Sausage Links
- Grilled Ham
- Applewood Smoked Bacon

Dessert

- Gluten-Free Chocolate Chip Pizookie

Alcoholic Beverages

- Berry Burst Cider
- Wyder's Pear Cider
- Redbridge Beer

Buffalo Wild Wings

Hand Spun Wings

- Traditional Chicken Wings

Tenders

- Naked Tenders (with or without Grill Seasoning)

Wing Sauces

- Sweet BBQ
- Mild Teriyaki
- Mild
- Parmesan Garlic
- Medium
- Honey BBQ
- Honey Mustard
- Spicy Garlic
- Caribbean Jerk
- Hot
- Mango Habanero
- Wild
- Blazin
- Cajun
- Desert Heat
- Buffalo
- Salt and Vinegar

- Chipotle
- Lemon Pepper
- Jammin Jalapeño

Shareables

- Ultimate Nachos
- Ultimate Nachos with Chicken
- Corn Tortilla Chips with Red Salsa
- Chili Con Queso with Corn Tortilla Chips

Sides

- French Fries
- Buffalo Chips
- Coleslaw
- Veggie Boat with Fat Free Ranch
- Wild Fries

Sandwiches

Without the Bun

- Pulled Pork
- Grilled Chicken Breast
- Burger Patty

Savory Salads

- Honey BBQ Chicken Salad with Cheese

Dressings and Sauces

- Bleu Cheese Dressing
- Ranch Dressing
- SW Ranch Dressing
- BBQ Ranch Dressing
- Fat Free Ranch

- Light Balsamic
- Light French
- Marinara Sauce
- Queso Cheese Sauce
- Chili
- Salsa Red
- Pico De Gallo
- Light Caesar Dressing
- Tartar Sauce
- Spicy Brown Mustard
- Cocktail Sauce

Desserts

- Ice Cream with Chocolate or Caramel Sauce

Kid's Meal

- Kid's Naked Tenders with Grilled Seasoning
- Kid's Traditional Wings
- French Fries

Cheeseburger in Paradise

For all sandwiches, be sure to order a GLUTEN FREE BUN!

First Wave aka Appetizers

- Black Angus Sliders without buns
- Loaded Chips

Sunset Salads and Soups

- Calypso Chicken Salad with grilled Chicken
- Son of a Sailor Salad

- Costa Rican Steak Salad without wontons

Paradise Specialties

- BBQ Ribs
- St. Barts Cirtus Chicken without Island Rice or Teriyaki Broccoli
- Parrot Beach Salmon without Island Rice or Teriyaki Broccoli

Cheeseburgers in Paradise

"We are proud to serve our New Gluten Free Bun for any of our burgers for 1.00 extra. A turkey and Veggie Burger can be substituted at no additional cost (Both are gluten free)." – Cheeseburger in Paradise

- Bacon Cheddar Burger
- Baja Burger
- Mini-Cheeseburgers without buns
- BBQ Bacon Burger
- All-American Beach Burger
- Black Angus Beef Burger

Surfside Sandwiches

- BBQ Chicken Sandwich with gluten free bun
- Fish Sandwich with gluten free bun

Sides

- French fried potatoes
- Vegetable of the day
- Coleslaw

Little Parakeets aka Kids Menu

Includes a choice of a beverage (soda, milk, or fresh parakeet punch) and a choice of a side (French fried potatoes, coleslaw, or mandarin oranges).

- Mini-Cheeseburgers without buns
- Grilled Chicken Breast
- BBQ Ribs
- Grilled Flame Steak

Sensuous Treats

- Copa Banana without Nilla Wafers
- Lil' Pirates Treat without Oreo cookie crumbles

Tiki Bar Favorites

- C.I.P Cocktail
- Blackberry Sangria
- House Piña Colada
- Pink Flamingo Rita
- Tropical Island Tea
- Red Bridge

Non-Alcoholic Beverages

- Hand-Dipped Milkshakes
- Island Paradise
- Jamaican Root Beer Float
- Surfside Sodas
- Flavored Iced Tea: Peach, Mango, Pomegranate, Raspberry and Blueberry

Other Drinks

- Strawberry Lemonade
- Island Lemonade
- Lemonade Iced Tea
- Brewed Iced Tea

- Freshly Brewed Coffee

Chili's

Soups

- Loaded Baked Potato
- Southwest Chicken and Sausage without tortilla strips

Salads

Listed without any salad dressings and croutons.

- Caribbean Salad with chicken or shrimp
- Chicken Caesar Salad
- House Salad
- Sante Fe Chicken Salad without tortilla strips

Salad Dressings

- Avocado-Ranch
- Bleu Cheese,
- Citrus-Balsamic Vinaigrette
- Honey Lime Dressing
- Honey Lime Vinaigrette
- Honey Mustard
- Low-Fat Ranch
- Non-Fat Honey Mustard
- Ranch

Sides

- Black Bean
- Coleslaw
- Corn Kernels

- Loaded Mashed Potatoes
- Mandarin Oranges
- Mashed Potatoes without Gravy
- Steamed Broccoli
- Sweet Corn on the Cobb

Slow Smoked In-House Ribs

- Memphis Dry Rub
- Original

Lighter Choices

- Classic Sirloin
- Grilled Chicken Salad
- Grilled Salmon
- Margarita Grilled Chicken without tortilla strips

Steaks

Be sure to get these steaks without the Garlic Toast.

- Classic Ribeye
- Classic Sirloin

Steak Toppers

- Sautéed Mushrooms
- Spicy Garlic and Lime Grilled Shrimp
- Chicken and Seafood
- Grilled Salmon with garlic and herbs
- Monterrey chicken

Burgers

Without buns, fries, onion strings, and tortilla strips

- Classic Bacon Burger

- Guacamole Burger without roasted pepper
- Jalapeno Smokehouse Burger
- Mushroom-Swiss Burger
- Oldtimer Burger
- Southern Smokehouse Burger

Pepper Pals

Order without buns

- Grilled Chicken Platter
- Grilled Chicken Sandwich
- Little Mouth Cheeseburger

Sauces and Extras

- Ancho-Chile Ranch
- Avocado Slices
- Bacon
- Guacamole
- Mixed Cheese
- Original BBQ
- Pico de Gallo
- Salsa
- Sautéed Mushrooms
- Sour Cream

Sweet Temptations

- Chocolate Shake

Daily Grill

Starters

- Shrimp Cocktail

- Seared Rare Ahi Tuna
- Trio of Hummus

Soup and Salads

- Manhattan Clam Chowder
- Mixed Green Salad
- Daily Grill Cobb Salad
- Charbroiled Chicken Caesar Salad
- Gazpacho
- The Grill Chopped Salad
- Grilled Lime Chicken Salad

Fresh Seafood

- Charbroiled Salmon
- Charbroiled Trout
- Cedar Plant Salmon
- Blackened Tilapia

DG Classics

- Filet Mignon
- New York Pepper Steak
- Double Cut Pork Chop
- Grilled Herb Chicken Breasts
- Pan Seared Chicken Piccata
- Grilled Vegetable Plate

Sides and Sauces

- Red Skin Mashed Potatoes
- Sautéed Spinach
- Baked Potato
- Herbed Brown Rice
- Steamed Spinach
- Grilled Asparagus

- Carrots
- Broccoli
- Lemon Butter Sauce
- Beurre Blanc Sauce
- Salsa Fresca
- Pomodoro Sauce

Desserts

- Sorbet and Berries
- All Natural Vanilla Ice Cream

Glory Days Grill

Wings (the sauces)

- Buffalo Style Medium
- Chi Chili
- Glory Wings made with Glory Days Grilling Sauce
- Old Bay
- Naked
- BBQ

Burgers and Sandwiches

Be sure to order these burgers and sandwiches without the bun

- The All American Burger
- Cheeseburger Trifecta
- Bacon and Cheddar Burger
- Swiss/Mushroom/Onion Burger without grilled onions
- Turkey Burger
- Hall of Fame Prime Cheeseburger
- The Glory Burger without onion straws
- Pigskin Burger without onion straws

- Hogettes BBQ Pork Sandwich
- Grilled Chicken Sandwich

Entrees

- Grilled Prime Rib with no grilled onions
- Grilled Shrimp Platter
- 10 Spice Chicken
- BBQ Ribs without cornbread
- Ribs and Grilled Shrimps
- Ribs and Wings
- Seared Tilapia
- BBQ Flat Iron Combo
- Fresh Grilled Salmon
- Buffalo Flat Iron Combo with no croutons
- New Orleans Flat Iron Combo with no croutons
- Glory Days Flat Iron Steak with no onions

Kids

- Hamburger or cheeseburger sliders with no bun
- Grilled Chicken strips
- BBQ ribs with no cornbread
- Side Toss Salad

Salads

Be sure to not order croutons

- Toss Salad
- BBQ Chicken
- Grilled Salmon
- Southwest BBQ Chopped Salad

Sides

- Seasoned fries
- Parsley pedskin potatoes

- Fresh seasonal vegetables
- Creamy coleslaw
- Sweet potato fries
- Side tossed salad request no croutons

Desserts

- Petit chocolate torte
- Hot fudge sundae

Ground Round Grill and Bar

Salads

- Grilled Chicken Club with honey mustard dressing
- Grilled Chicken and Spinach with raspberry balsamic vinaigrette

Salad Dressings

- Ranch
- French
- Honey Mustard
- Raspberry Vinaigrette
- Italian
- Caesar
- Thousand Island
- Bleu Cheese

Light Classics

- Stuffed Baked Potato and Salad with a choice of these toppings: buffalo, chicken ranch, broccoli cheese, or bacon cheese

Fresh Bunless Burgers

Be sure to order these burgers without any buns

- The Ground Rounder
- Bruschetta Burger

Ribs

- BBQ Baby Back Ribs

Chicken

- Boneless Chicken Dinner
- Steak
- Choice-Center Cut Sirloin
- Choice 12 oz NY Strip

Seafood

- Haddock baked or broiled without breadcrumbs
- Grilled Salmon without garlic toast

Add Ons and Sides

- Half rack of ribs
- Grilled chicken
- Baked Potato
- House Vegetable
- Broccoli
- Mashed Red Skin Potatoes
- House or Caesar Salad with no croutons
- Grilled Asparagus

Green Mill

Hand Made Burger

Made with Udi's gluten free buns and without onion rings or haystack onions.

- Mushroom swiss
- Summit bacon
- Four cheese bacon
- Western mill
- Cheeseburger
- Bacon jalapeno with Havarti
- Veggie burger

Sensational Salads

- Cilantro Lime Shrimp Salad
- Pecan Craisin Spinach Salad with non-marinated chicken
- Cobb Salad with Chicken with non-marinated chicken
- All Salad dressings except Ginger Soy

Pizza

Order pizza with Udi's gluten free crust

- Gluten free pizza

Hooters

For a place called Hooters, you'd expect everything to be big. [naughty joke]

But that can't be said about the Hooter's gluten free menu.

Salads

Order without croutons and bleu cheese

- Side Caesar Salad
- Side Entrée Salad
- Entrée Garden Salad
- Entrée Caesar Salad

Sandwiches & Entrées

All sandwiches should be ordered without bun or bread

- Big Fish Grilled Sandwich: Should be prepared without season
- Gourmet Hot Dog: Gluten-free toppings include cheddar cheese, diced onions, and relish
- Grilled Chicken Sandwich: Should be prepared without any seasoning
- Hooters Burger: Gluten free toppings include Swiss and cheddar cheese, bacon, and sautéed vegetables which have been prepared without seasoning

Seafood

Be sure to request no saltine crackers

- Oysters (raw)
- Crab Legs: Should be prepared without shrimp boil
- Steam Clams
- Steamed Shrimp: Should be prepared without shrimp boil

Sides

- Potato Salad
- Coleslaw
- Baked Beans

- Side Salad
- Carrot and Celery

Iron Hill Brewery and Restaurant

Salad Starters

- Mesclun Salad
- Red Quinoa Salad
- Red Beet and Goat Cheese Salad
- Caesar Salad
- Garden Salad

Big Salads

- Grilled North Atlantic Salmon Salad, ordered without Salmon
- Fajita Spiced Chicken Salad without Chicken
- Cabo Shrimp Salad without Shrimp

Appetizers

- Brabant Mussels
- Voodoo Shrimp

Shared Plates

- Hummus
- Baked Chicken Wings

8 oz Beef Burgers

Order with without bread

- Brewski Burger
- Santa Fe Burger

- Slammin Jammin Burger
- Cheeseburger

Sandwiches

Order with without bread

- Turkey Burger
- House Smoked Pork
- Grilled Chicken
- Portobello Mushroom Sandwich
- Pecan Chicken Salad

Healthy Selections

- Fajita Spiced Chicken Breast
- Moroccan Salmon
- Pan Roasted Beef Tenderloin Medallion

Entrees

- Petite Filet Mignon
- Beef Tenderloin Medallions Stroganoff
- Shrimp, Catfish, Andouille, Red Beans and Rice
- Char-Grilled Flat Iron Steak

Desserts

- Flourless chocolate torte

Not Your Average Joe's

According to Joe's, every meal starts with a gluten free version of their legendary bread and dip.

Appetizers

- Thai Chicken Lettuce Wraps
- House Made Guacamole

Entree Salads

- Cobb
- Waldorf
- Ahi Tuna
- Chicken Mona Lisa
- House Salad

Salad Dressings

- Low-cal zinfandel
- Orange-sesame vinaigrette
- Creamy ranch
- Balsamic vinaigrette
- Raspberry vinaigrette

horseradish-mustard

Burgers & Sandwiches

On gluten free buns/rolls

- Backyard Burger
- House Roasted Turkey BLT
- Grilled Chicken Sandwich

Entrees

- Vietnamese Flounder
- Rosemary Skewered Scallops
- Baked Fresh Haddock
- Chicken Piccata
- Chicken Breast
- Grilled Salmon
- Great Hill Sirloin Wedge
- Mediterranean Chicken
- Grilled Turkey Kabob

Kids Menu

- Grilled Chicken Breast
- Grilled Salmon
- Classic Burger on a gluten free roll

Sides

- Sautéed green beans
- roasted vegetables
- Garlic mashed potatoes
- Grilled asparagus

Dessert

- Passion Fruit Sorbet

Ruby Tuesday

Be sure request no Garlic Cheese Biscuits to be served.

Garden Fresh Salads

- Grilled Chicken Salad: No croutons

Create Your Own Garden Bar with toppings:

- Sliced tomatoes, edamame, green peas, diced eggs, parmesan cheese, bacon bits, diced ham, black olives, sunflower seeds

Dressings:

- Thousand Island, Balsamic Vinaigrette, Zesty Italian, Ranch, Lite Ranch, Honey Mustard, Olive Oil, and Vinegar

Premium Seafood

- New Orleans Seafood without parmesan cream sauce
- Blackened Tilapia with Mango Salsa
- Grilled Salmon
- Creole Catch
- Jumbo Skewered Shrimp

Fresh All-Natural Chicken

- Chicken Fresco without lemon-butter sauce
- Chicken Bella without Parmesan cream sauce
- Barbecue Grilled Chicken without Boston barbecue sauce
- Chicken Trio with no lemon-butter sauce on the Chicken Fresco, no Parmesan cream sauce on the Chicken Bella, and no rice pilaf

Steakhouse Steaks

- Asiago Peppercorn Sirloin without Parmesan cream sauce
- Top Sirloin
- Chef's Cut Sirloin
- Petite Sirloin and Lobster Tail
- Petite Sirloin

- Rib Eye

Pasta Classics

- Spaghetti Squash Marinara

Fork-Tender Ribs

No Coconut-Crusted Shrimp or Louisiana Fried Shrimp add-on

- Memphis Dry Rub Baby Back Ribs

Fresh. Fresh. Sides

- Fresh grilled zucchini
- Sugar snap peas
- Fresh steamed broccoli
- Fresh grilled green beans
- Roasted spaghetti squash
- Fresh baked potato
- White cheddar mashed potatoes
- Loaded baked potato
- Fresh grilled asparagus
- Diced apples (kid's menu)
- Grapes (kid's menu)
- Sliced tomatoes with balsamic vinaigrette

Fresh Lunch Combinations (Mon-Fri until 3 p.m.)

- Veggie Trio and Garden Bar

Petite Lunch Plates (Mon-Fri until 3 p.m.)

- Jumbo Shrimp Scampi
- Creole Catch
- Sliced Sirloin
- Chicken Fresco without lemon-butter sauce

Fresh Handcrafted Burgers

No bun and no French fries

- Ruby's Classic Burger
- Classic Cheeseburger
- Bacon Cheeseburger
- Smokehouse Burger: no onion rings or barbecue sauce
- Triple Prime Burger
- Triple Prime Cheddar Burger
- Triple Prime Bacon Cheddar Burger
- Avocado Grilled Chicken Sandwich
- Turkey Burger
- Avocado Turkey Burger

Kid's Menu

- Beef Mini Burgers without the bun
- Grilled Chicken
- Chop Steak

Brunch

No brunch potatoes

- Western Omelet: Order with no Hollandaise sauce

Steak and Eggs

Kid's Brunch

No brunch potatoes

- Eggscellent Combo

Shane's Rib Shack

Plates

- Pork
- Barbecue Chicken
- Half Chicken
- Whole Chicken
- Half Rack Ribs
- Full Rack Ribs
- Beef Brisket
- Grilled Chicken Tenders

Salads

- The Shack (Pork or Chicken)
- Grilled Chicken
- Beef Brisket

Barbecue Sauce

- Shane's Original Barbecue Sauce

Sides

- Baked Beans
- Coles Slaw
- Corn on the Cob
- Green Beans
- Side Salads
- Chips

Smokey Bones

Firestarters

- Fire Stix
- Smoked Wings
- Salsa
- Firecracker Shrimp with no Pretzel

Salads and Soups

- Side Green Salad with no croutons
- Side Caesar Salad
- Charbroiled Caesar Salad
- Cobb Salad
- Nutty Grilled Chicken Salad
- All dressings

Fire Grilled Steak

- Top Sirloin Steak with no chipotle marinade
- NY Strip Steak
- Pork Tenderloin with Chipotle BBQ Glaze
- All toppings except mushroom sauce

Chicken and Seafood

- BBQ Chicken
- Grilled Chicken Breast
- Flamed Seared Salmon without sauce

Ribs

- Smoked St Louis Style Ribs
- Baby Back Ribs
- Smoked Beef Brisket
- Sliced Smoke Turkey Breast

Sides

- French Fries (Fried in Canola)
- Coleslaw
- Broccoli
- Apples
- Mashed Potatoes without gravy
- Loaded Mashed Potatoes
- Baked Potato
- Loaded Baked Potato

Ted's Montana Grill

Starters

- Grilled Shrimp without bread

Salads

- Balsamic Bleu Steak without crispy fried onion straws
- Classic Caesar: Chicken, Cedar plank salmon, or grilled shrimo
- Big Sky Grilled: Chicken, beef burger, bison burger, or cedar plank salmon
- Ted's Chopped
- Iceberg Wedge
- House
- Classic Caesar Side

Salad Dressings

Be sure to request for no croutons

- "Eggless" Caesar
- Honey Mustard

- Basil Vinaigrette
- Bleu Cheese
- Olive Oil
- Red Wine Vinegar
- Thousand Island

Classics

Order without yeast roll

- Cedar Plank Salmon
- Salt-And-Pepper Trout
- Prime Rib without au juis
- Bison or Beef Tenderloin Filet
- Bison Kansas City Strip Steak
- Bison or Beef Delmonico
- Roast Turkey without dressing and gravy

Sides

- Asparagus
- Vine-Ripened Tomatoes
- Sweet Potato
- Roasted Broccoli
- Cole Slaw
- Baked Potato
- Buttered Carrots
- French Cut Fries
- Garlic Mashed Potatoes: without gravy

Burgers

Order without the bun

Choose from naturally raised bison or certified angus beef or all natural chicken.

- Naked

- Cheese
- Ted's Bacon Cheeseburger
- Avalon
- Peppercorn
- George's Cadillac
- Blue Creek
- Vermejo
- Swiss and Mushroom
- America's Cup
- Canyon Creek
- Skinny Dip
- Kitchen Sink

Kids' Menu

- Bar Non Sliders without bun
- Cedar Plank Salmon
- Steak and Fries

Desserts

- Häagen-Dazs Ice Cream
- Hand-Made Shakes
- Floats: Coke, ICB Rootbeer

Wildfire Grill

Appetizers

- Baked Fresh Onion Soup
- Chicken and Portobello Mushroom Skewers
- Baked Goat Cheese
- Spinach and Artichoke Fondue
- Wildfire Mussels
- Jumbo Shrimp Cocktail

- Roasted Sea Scallop Skewers

Pizza

Made with a gluten free crust

- Fresh Mozzarella Pizza
- Chicken Sausage Pizza
- Grilled Pepperoni Pizza

Salads

- House Salad Bowl
- Caesar
- Spinach
- Greek
- Roasted Bee and Goat Cheese
- Wildfire Chopped Salad
- Grilled Chicken Wildorf Salad
- Grilled Steak and Blue Cheese
- Mediterranean Shrimp Salad

Pasta

Pasta is made from brown rice

- Penne and Wood Roasted Vegetables
- Shrimp and Penne

Steak, Chops, and Prime Rib

- Petit Filet Mignon
- Filet Mignon
- High Plains Bison Beef
- Wildfire Bone In Filet
- Pork Chops
- Broiled Prime Sirloin Steak
- Basil Haydens Bourbon Tenderloin Tips

- Roumanian Skirt Steak
- New York Steaj
- Lamb Porterhouse Chops
- Bone In Rib Eye
- Porterhouse
- Classic Surf and Turf
- Primte Rib

Wildfire Sauces

- Bearnaise
- Peppercorn
- Shallot Balsamic

Fresh Fish and Seafood

- Cedar Planked Salmon
- Swordfish London Broil
- Tuna Steak Teriyaki
- Whole Roasted Sea Bass
- Macadamia Nut Crusted Halibut

Chicken and Barbecue

- Spit Roasted Half Chicken
- Barbecued Chicken
- Lemon Pepper Chicken Breasts
- Chicken Moreno
- Barbecued Baby Back Ribs
- Half Long Island Duck

Prime Burgers and Sandwiches

Served on a homemade gluten free bun

- Thick Prime Angus Burger
- Charbroiled Cheeseburger
- Handmade Black Bean

- All Natural Turkey Burger
- High Plains Bison Burger Deluxe
- Grilled Chicken Club
- Prime Rib French Dip
- Tenderloin Steak Sandwich
- Classic BLT Club
- Sliced Turkey Sandwich
- Grilled Buffalo Chicken Sandwich
- Blackened Salmon Sandwich

Sides

- Redskin Mashed Potatoes
- Fresh Broccoli
- Five Grain Wild Rice
- Balsamic Roasted Vegetables
- Macaroni and Cheese
- Au Gratin Potatoes
- Giant Baked Idaho Potato
- BBQ Rubbed Sweet Potato
- Wood Roasted Mushroom Caps
- Cheddar Double Stuffed Potato

Desserts

- Flourless Chocolate Cake
- Chocolate Chip Cookies
- Fresh Berries
- Vanilla Ice Cream Sundae

Sandwiches, Deli, & Salads

If you're ever in the mood for a hoagie, submarine sandwich, Panini, or customized salad, this is your section.

Au Bon Pain

Entrées

- Mayan Chicken Harvest Rice Bowl with brown or white rice

Salad

- BBQ Beef Salad
- Egg and Cucumber Salad
- Potato Bacon Salad
- Red Bliss Potato Salad
- Tomato and Cucumber Salad
- Tomato, Green Bean and Almond Salad
- Tuna Salad
- Watermelon and Feta Salad
- Chef's Salad
- Greek Salad
- Mediterranean Chicken Salad

Dressings, Sauces, and Spreads

- All sauces, condiments, and spreads

Soup

- Black Bean Soup
- Curried Rice and Lentil Soup
- Fresh Moroccan Tomato Lentil
- Garden Vegetable

- Gazpach
- Portuguese Kale
- Potato Cheese
- Southwest Tortilla
- Beef Chili
- Vegetarian Chili
- Tuscan white bean

Sides

- White rice
- Brown rice
- Roasted Potatoes
- Sausage with Pepper and Onions
- Scrambled Eggs
- Oatmeal
- Apple Cinnamon Oatmeal
- Hummus and Cucumber Portion
- Mozzarella and Tomato Portion
- Turkey, Asparagus, Cranberry, Chutney and Gorgonzola Portion

Snacks and Dessert

- All yogurts
- Chocolate Covered Strawberry
- Dark Chocolate Covered Raisins
- Fresh Grapes
- Fresh Pineapples
- Fresh Watermelon
- Fruit Cup
- Mixed Nuts
- Muesli
- Sugar Free Cinnamon Buttons
- Turkish Apricots
- Apples, Blue Cheese and Cranberries Portion

Blimpie

Individual Menu Items

- Bacon
- Buffalo Chicken
- Cappacola
- Grilled Chicken Strips
- Corned Beef
- Ham
- Pastrami
- Pepperoni
- Philly Steak & Onion
- Prosciuttini
- Roast Beef
- Salami
- Seafood Salad
- Tuna
- Turkey
- American Yellow & White
- Smoked Cheddar
- Shredded Mild Cheddar
- Shredded Parmesan
- Provolone
- Swiss

Salads

- Antipasto
- Buffalo Chicken
- Chef
- Chicken Caesar
- Tuna
- Ultimate Club
- Garden
- Cole Slaw

- Northwest Potato
- Potato

Soups

- Captain's Corn Chowder
- Cream of Broccoli with Cheese
- Cream of Potato
- Grande Chili with Bean & Beef X
- Pilgrim Turkey Vegetables with Rice

Dressings and Sauces

- All sauces and dressings

Charley's Grilled Subs

Entrées without Toasted Bun

- Philly Cheesesteak
- Philly Steak Deluxe
- BBQ Cheddar
- Bacon 3 Cheese
- Sicilian Steak
- Mushroom Swiss Steak
- Philly Steak and Bleu
- Philly Chicken
- Chicken California
- Chicken Buffalo
- Chicken Teriyaki
- Chicken Cordon Bleu
- Chicken Bacon Club
- Turkey Cheddar Melt
- Philly Ham and Swiss
- Italian Deli

- Philly Veggie

Sides

NOTE: All fries should be avoided by anyone who is Celiac or has a gluten sensitivity. Since the fries are cooked in the same baskets as the breaded chicken fingers found on the kid's menu, there is a high chance of cross contamination.

- Fries
- Ranch Bacon Fries
- Cheddar Bacon Fries
- Cheddar Fries
- Ultimate fries

Salad

- Grilled Chicken Salad
- Chicken Teriyaki Salad
- Buffalo Chicken Salad
- Grilled Steak Salad
- Fresh Garden Salad

Breakfast

- Two eggs scrambled
- Ham Omelet
- Bacon Omelet
- Sausage Omelet
- Veggie Omelet
- Western Omelet
- Egg and Cheese Sandwich
- Bacon, Egg and Cheese Sandwich
- Sausage, Egg and Cheese Sandwich
- Steak, Egg and Cheese Sandwich
- Hash Browns

Cousins Sub Sandwiches

Meats

- Ham
- Turkey Breast
- Chicken Breast
- Bacon (BLT)

Greens

- Gourmet Garden
- Gourmet Garden Salad with Chicken
- Turkey Bacon Delight
- Almond Berry Chicken

Soups

- Cheddar Cauliflower
- Cheddar Cheese
- Cream of Broccoli with Cheese
- Chili
- Cream of Potato

Sweets

- Peanut Butter Crisp Bar

Extra Toppings, Sauces, and Dressings

- Bacon Slices
- BBQ Ranch
- BBQ Sauce
- Cheese (cheddar, provolone, sharp, swiss)
- Cucumber slices
- Fat Free Raspberry Vinaigrette
- Green Peppers

- Hot Pepper Relish
- Jalapeno Slices
- Lettuce
- Marinara Sauce
- Mayonnaise
- Mushroom
- Mustard (brown spicy or yellow)
- Olives
- Onions
- Pepperoncini (sliced or unsliced)
- Pickle slices
- Ranch Dressing
- Red Wine Vinegar
- Salad Oil
- Tomatoes

Erbert and Gerbert's

Erbert and Gerbert's has gluten free versions of 3 of their sandwiches which are prepared using dedicated equipment to avoid any cross contamination. Also, their gluten free buns are designed by Udi's and certified by the GFCO.

Certified Gluten Free Sandwiches

- The Bone Billy
- The Comet Morehouse
- The Jacob Bluefinger

Subs

Be sure to request the gluten free buns. Erbert and Gerbert's can't certify these subs to be gluten free.

- Pompeii

- Titan
- Erupter
- Spartan
- Quatro
- Comet Candy
- Flash
- Narmer
- Girf
- Tullius
- Shortcake
- Giza
- Geeter
- Bone Billy
- Comet Morehouse
- Halleys Comet
- Jacob Bluefinger
- Cally
- Tappy
- Bornk
- Pudder

Soups

Be sure to request the certified gluten free soups.

- Cheddar Cheese & Broccoli
- Cheesy Asparagus
- French Onion

Fresh to Order

Salads

- Asian with no noodles
- Blue Cheese Fig Salad

- Caesar Salad with no croutons
- Club
- Chopped Wedge
- Market
- Southwestern
- Spinach
- Mediterranean

Salad Dressings

- Blue Cheese,
- Evo & Aged Balsamic
- Honey Mustard,
- Balsamic Vinaigrette
- Ranch
- Lemon and Herbs

Add-Ons for Salads

- Un-Crusted Grilled Tuna Steak
- Tofu with no dressing
- Un-Marinated Salmon
- Un-Marinated Grilled Chicken Tenders

Long Plates

- Brown Sugar Roasted Pork Loin
- Salmon Entree with no sauce, seasoning or bread
- Un-Marinated Grilled Chicken Breast

Sides

- Garlic Mashed Potatoes
- Grilled Vegetables
- Sweet Mashed Potatoes

Sauces

- Orange Chili Glaze
- Apricot Chutney

Jason's Deli

Build Your Own Sandwich

- Gluten-free bread
- Hot pastrami
- Hot corned beef
- Roast beef
- Oven roasted turkey breast
- Smoked turkey breast
- Premium ham
- Chicken salad made with almonds & pineapple
- Tuna salad
- Hard salami
- Natural grilled chicken breast
- Yellow mustard
- Organic stone ground mustard
- Mayonnaise
- Smoked red pepper-cilantro aioli
- Leo's Italian dressing
- Balsamic Vinegar (bottle)
- Extra virgin olive oil
- Lettuce
- Tomato
- Organic field greens
- Organic spinach
- Purple onion rings
- Italian peppers
- Our family recipe pico de gallo

- Our family recipe guacamole
- Sliced avocado
- Oven roasted herb tomatoes
- Swiss
- American
- Cheddar
- Jalapeño pepper jack
- Provolone

Soups

- Vegetarian Tomato Basil
- Organic Vegetable Soup
- Fire-Roasted Tortilla
- Red Beans & Rice with sausage

Salads and Salad Bar Toppings

- Big Chef
- Nutty Mixed Up Salad
- Chicken Club Salad
- Lettuce
- Organic field greens
- Organic spinach
- Cauliflower
- Grape tomatoes
- Broccoli
- Mushrooms
- Organic baby carrots
- Red bell pepper rings
- Yellow bell pepper rings
- Purple onion rings
- Cucumber slices
- Sprouts
- Green olives
- Kalamata olives
- Artichokes

- Italian peppers
- Hard boiled eggs
- Bacon bits
- Organic apple slices
- Mixed fruit and yogurt
- Cottage cheese
- Feta
- Shredded asiago
- Shredded cheddar
- Roasted red pepper hummus
- American potato salad
- Coleslaw
- Walnut cranberry trail mix
- Chocolate mousse

Dressings

- Bleu Cheese
- Low fat Honey Mustard
- Our family recipe Ranch
- Low fat Ranch
- Leo's Italian
- Organic Raspberry Vinaigrette
- Creamy Caesar
- Thousand Island
- Organic Country French
- Extra Virgin Olive Oil (bottle)
- Organic Balsamic Vinegar

Potatoes

- Texas Style Spud
- Pollo Mexicano
- The Plain Jane

Sides

- Chips or baked chips & pickle
- Organic blue corn tortilla chips & salsa
- Organic blue corn tortilla chips &
- Roasted red pepper hummus
- Organic blue corn tortilla chips &guacamole
- American potato salad
- Steamed veggies
- Fresh fruit & creamy fruit dip

Desserts

- Chocolate or vanilla ice cream with no cone
- Chocolate syrup topping

Kid's Menu

- Grilled Cheese on gluten-free bread
- Hot dog on gluten-free bun
- Organic Peanut Butter and Jelly on gluten-free bread
- Ham and Cheese on gluten-free bread
- Turkey and Cheese on gluten-free bread

Panera Bread

Below is a listing of Panera Bread's hidden menu, which is all gluten free.

Breakfast

- Power Breakfast Egg White Bowl with Roasted Turkey
- Power Breakfast Egg Bowl with Steak

Lunch and Dinner

- Power Mediterranean Chicken Salad
- Power Mediterranean Roasted Turkey Salad

- Power Chicken Hummus Bowl
- Power Steak Lettuce Wraps

Below is a listing of Panera Bread's normal menu with gluten free options.

Salads

- Greek Salad Caesar Salad without croutons
- Grilled Chicken
- Caesar Salad without croutons
- Asian Sesame Chicken Salad without Won Ton noodles
- Classic Cafe Salad
- Fuji Apple Chicken Salad
- Chopped Chicken Cobb Salad
- Strawberry Poppyseed Chicken Salad
- Tomato and Mozzarella Salad without croutons
- BBQ Chopped Chicken Salad
- Fruit Cup – Watermelon
- Seasonal Mixed Fruit Cup

Salad Dressings

- Balsamic Vinaigrette
- Caesar
- Greek
- Poppyseed Dressing
- Asian Sesame Vinaigrette
- White Balsamic Vinaigrette
- BBQ Ranch
- Light Buttermilk Ranch

Soups

- Low Fat Vegetarian Black Bean
- Creamy Tomato without croutons

Beverages

- Tea, regular and Chai Tea
- All lattes & Frozen beverages
- Low-fat Strawberry Smoothie
- Low-Fat Black Cherry Smoothie
- Low-Fat Mango Smoothie
- Low-fat Wild Berry Smoothie
- Frozen Strawberry Lemonade
- Frozen Lemonade
- Hot Chocolate

Sides

- Panera Bread Potato Chips

Potbelly Sandwiches

Meats and Other Sandwich "Main Stuff"

- Turkey Breast
- Italian Meat (Salami, Capicolla, Mortadello, Pepperoni)
- Smoked Ham
- Tuna Salad
- Grilled Chicken
- Roast Beef
- Hummus
- Marinara
- Peanut Butter
- Jelly
- Bacon

Cheese

- Swiss

- Provolone
- Cheddar
- Blue Cheese
- Feta

Sandwich Toppings

- Mayo
- Mustard
- Hot Peppers
- Iceberg Lettuce
- Tomatoes
- Onions
- Pickles
- Oil
- Roasted Red Peppers
- Artichokes
- Italian Seasonings

Salad Toppings

- Romaine, Iceberg Lettuce
- Apples
- Candied Walnuts
- Cucumbers
- Cherry Tomatoes
- Grapes
- Hard Boiled Egg
- Blue Cheese
- Chick Peas

Salad Dressings

- Buttermilk Ranch
- Potbelly Vinaigrette
- Non-Fat Vinaigrette
- Balsamic Vinaigrette

Soups

- Garden Vegetable
- Spicy Black Bean and Roasted Tomato

Fresh To Go

- Hard Boiled Egg 2 Pack
- Yogurt Parfait
- Seasonal Fruit
- Chicken Salad Square Meal
- Tuna Salad Square Meal
- Tomato Cucumber Salad
- Chicken Salad Salad
- Wreck Salad
- Side Salads
- Coleslaw
- Potato Salad

Shakes and Smoothies

Be sure to request no butter cookie.

- Vanilla
- Chocolate
- Coffee
- Banana
- Strawberry
- Mixed Berry

Breakfast Items Only

- Sausage
- Egg Patties

Quiznos

Meats and Proteins

- Bacon
- Capicola
- Chicken
- Hard Boiled Eggs
- Honey Ham
- Pepperoni
- Pork
- Roasted Turkey
- Salami
- Sausage Patty
- Scrambled Egg Patty
- Tuna

Cheese

- Blue Cheese Crumbles
- Italian 3-Cheese Blend
- Cheddar
- Mozzarella
- Swiss

Sauces and Dressings

- Acai Vinaigrette
- Basil Pesto
- Buttermilk Ranch
- Chipotle Mayonnaise
- County BBQ
- Creamy Horseradish
- Fat Free Balsamic
- Four Pepper Chili Sauce
- Guacamole
- Honey Bourbon Mustard

- Honey French
- Honey Mustard
- Lite Mayonnaise
- Marinara Sauce
- Peppercorn Sauce
- Peppercorn Caesar
- Red Wine Vinaigrette
- Tzatziki
- Yellow Mustard
- Grille Sauce

Toppings and Extras

- Dried Cranberries
- Pepitas (Pumpkin Seeds)
- Seasonal Greens
- Apples
- Cucumbers
- Grapes
- Green Bell Pepper
- Mushrooms
- Red Onion
- Sauteed Mushrooms
- Sauteed Yellow Onion
- Shredded Lettuce
- Tomato
- Yellow Onion

Salads

- Peppercorn Caesar
- Harvest Chicken
- Honey Mustard
- Cobb

Runza

Soups

- Broccoli Cheese Soup

Salads

- Sweet Berry Chicken Salad with no dressing

Dressings and Sauces

- Fat Free Italian Dressing
- Jalapeño Ranch Dressing
- Ranch Dressing
- Fat Free Raspberry Vinaigrette Dressing
- Poppyseed Dressing
- Asian Dressing
- BBQ Sauce
- Honey Mustard

Sides

- French Onion Dip
- Mandarin Oranges
- Bacon Slices
- Mayo
- The Runza Way
- Applesauce

Desserts and Shakes

- Chocolate Sundae
- Caramel Sundae
- Turtle Sundae
- Vanilla Ice Cream in a Dish
- Chocolate Ice Cream in a Dish

- Swirl Ice Cream in a Dish
- Vanilla Shake
- Chocolate Shake
- Strawberry Shake
- Cappuccino Shake
- Cherry Slushy
- Blue Raspberry Slushy
- Grape Slushy
- Pepsi Slushy
- Mountain Dew Slushy

SaladWorks

Salads and Toppings

- Eggs/Egg Whites
- Fire Roasted Red Pepper
- Grated Parmesan
- Ham
- Mandarin Oranges
- Monterey Jack
- Mozzarella
- Olives
- Pepperoni
- Sun Dried Tomatoes
- Sunflower Seeds
- Swiss Cheese
- Tofu
- Tortilla Strips
- Tuna
- Turkey
- Walnuts
- Provolone Cheese
- Bacon

- Blue Cheese Crumbles
- Chicken
- Corn blend

Dressings

- Blue Cheese Dressing
- Dressing Creamy Italian
- Lite Ranch Dressing
- FF Balsamic Dressing
- FF Caesar Dressing
- FF Honey Dressing
- French Dressing
- Green Goddess Dressing
- Italian Vinaigrette Dressing
- Lite Raspberry Dressing
- Parm Peppercorn Dressing
- Ranch Dressing
- Russian Dressing
- Balsamic Vinaigrette Dressing
- Lemon Capri Dressing
- Yogurt Caesar Dressing
- Yogurt Italian Dressing

Soups

- Beef Chili
- Broccoli Cheddar
- Chicken Chili
- Chicken Tortilla

Smiling Moose

One of the best things about Smiling Moose is the fact that almost their entire menu has a gluten free alternative. So with that being said, be sure to request a gluten free bun for your sandwiches.

Hot Sandwiches

- The Mighty Mo!
- Parisian
- Hot Turkey Club
- Green Thumb

Cold Sandwiches

- Chicken or Tuna Salad
- The Sidecar
- Hippie Chick P
- Soups
- Cream of tomato basil
- Hearty Vegetable

Salads

- Ty Cobb

Salad Dressings

- Balsamic Vinaigrette
- Bleu Cheese
- Orange Rosemary
- Ranch

Breakfast

- The Morning Moose
- Jo's Morning

Subway

Although there currently isn't an official gluten free bun that you can get, Subways has been testing out gluten free sub rolls at select locations in the U.S. and Canada.

Meats

- Buffalo Chicken
- Chicken and Bacon Ranch
- Cold Cut Combo
- Ham (Black Forest)
- Italian BMT
- Oven Roasted Chicken with Chicken Strips
- Roast Beef
- Tuna
- Turkey Breast
- Turkey Breast and Ham
- Spicy Italian
- Subway Club
- Veggie Delight

Meat, Poultry, Seafood, and Eggs

- Bacon Strips
- Oven Roasted Chicken
- Chicken Strips (plain)
- Cold Cut Combo Meats
- Egg (Regular) Omelet
- Egg (White) Omelet
- Ham (Black Forest)
- Italian BMT® Meats
- Roast Beef
- Steak
- Tuna
- Turkey Breast

Cheese

- American Cheese
- Cheddar Cheese
- Monterey Cheddar Cheese, Shredded
- Mozzarella Cheese, Shredded
- Parmesan Cheese
- Pepper Jack Cheese
- Provolone Cheese
- Swiss Cheese

Condiments and Dressing

- Buffalo Sauce
- Chipotle Southwest Sauce
- Honey Mustard Sauce
- Light Mayonnaise/Regular Mayonnaise
- Mustard (Yellow and Deli Brown)
- Oil
- Ranch Dressing
- Red Wine Vinaigrette
- Sweet Onion Sauce (Contains Poppy Seeds)
- Vinegar

Vegetables

- Banana Peppers
- Jalapenos
- Olives
- Pickles
- Vegetables, Fresh

Ted's Hot Dogs

Be sure to request a gluten free hot dog or hamburger bun for your meal.

Hot Dogs

Request a gluten free hot dog bun by Udi's

- Regular
- Footlong
- Skinless
- All Beef Jumbo

Burgers

- *Request a gluten free hamburger bun by Udi's*
- Regular
- Jumbo
- Double
- Sausage
- Italian Sausage with Pepper and Onions
- Polish Sausage with Pepper and Onions

Sides

The french fries are naturally gluten free. However, since they are cooked in the same fryers as onion rings, which contain gluten.

- French Fries
- Potato Salad

Milkshakes

- Chocolate
- Vanilla
- Strawberry
- Loganberry

- Orange Cram Shake

Sauces, Toppings, and Condiments

- Ketchup
- Mustard
- Hot Sauce
- Relish
- Pickle
- Onion
- Lettuce
- Tomato
- Mayonnaise
- BBQ Sauce
- Sauerkraut
- Chili
- Cheese
- Peppers and Onions

Which Wich

Sandwiches

Be sure to order without bread

- Beef Cheesesteak
- Corned Beef
- Reuben
- Roast Beef
- Bacon and Egg
- Green Eggs and Ham
- Ham and Egg
- Sausage and Egg
- Veggies and Egg
- Buffalo Chicken

- Chicken
- Chicken Cordon Bleu
- Chicken Pesto
- Chicken Salad
- BLT
- Egg Salad
- BBQ Pork and Slaw
- Bac-Hammon
- Ham
- The Cuban
- The Hula
- Large Chicken Parm
- Large Grinder
- Large Muffuletta
- Large Pepperoni Pizzawich
- Siracha Tuna
- Tuna Salad
- Turkey Club
- Turkey Reuben
- Turkeywich
- The Wicked

Lettuce Bowl

- Combo Bowlwich
- Lettuce Bowlwich
- Spinach Bowlwich

Shakes

- Banana
- Chocolate
- Pineapple
- Strawberry
- Vanilla

Toppings

- 100 Island Dressing
- American Cheese
- Artichoke Hearts
- Avocado
- BBQ Sauce
- Bacon Balsamic Vinaigrette Dressing
- Banana Peppers
- Bell Peppers
- Black Olives
- Blue Cheese
- Buffalo Sauce
- Caprese
- Caramelized Onions
- Cheddar Cheese
- Cheez Whiz
- Coleslaw
- Crushed Red Pepper
- Cucumbers
- Deli Mustard
- Dijon Mustard
- Fat Free Italian Dressing
- Feta Cheese
- Garlic
- Honey Mustard
- Honey Mustard Dressing
- Horseradish Mayo
- Hot Pepper Mix
- Hummus
- Iceberg Lettuce
- Jalapeños
- Light Mayo
- Marinara Sauce
- Mozzarella Cheese
- Mushrooms

- Oil
- Olive Salad
- Oregano
- Parmesan Cheese
- Pepper
- Pepper Jack Cheese
- Pesto Sauce
- Pickles
- Provolone Cheese
- Ranch Dressing
- Red Onions
- Mayo
- Salt
- Sauerkraut
- Spicy Mayo
- Spicy Ranch Dressing
- Spinach
- Swiss Cheese
- Tomatoes
- Vinegar
- Yellow Mustard

Seafood

This section is for seafood lovers only. From grilled salmon to shrimp scampi, you'll be sure to find a filling gluten free seafood meal in this section.

Bonefish Grill

Salads

- Bonefish Caesar: Order without croutons.
- Bonefish House
- Grilled Salmon + Asparagus Salad:
- Florida Cobb Salad

Starters + Sharing

- Edamame
- Mussels Josephine
- Saucy Shrimp

Grilled Fish over wood-burning grill

- Dorado (Mahi Mahi)
- Chilean Sea Bass
- Atlantic Salmon
- Sea Scallops + Shrimp
- Snake River Rainbow Trout
- Longfin Tilapia
- Cold Water Lobster Tails

Signature Sauces for the Grilled Fish

- Mango Salsa
- Chimichurri
- Lemon Butter

Grilled Specialties over wood-burning grill

- Lily's Chicken
- Filet Mignon USDA Choice
- "The Angler's Steak" Special

Fresh Vegetable Sides

- Garlic Whipped Potatoes Steamed Broccoli
- Herbed Jasmine Rice Steamed Asparagus
- French Green Beans (Haricot Verts)
- Vegetable Medley

All entrées are served with a fresh seasonal vegetable plus your choice of one side item

Desserts

- Macadamia Nut Brownie
- Crème Brûlée

Adult Beverages

- All martinis, rocks and wines are gluten free.

Bubba Gump Shrimp Co

Many of Bubba Gump Shrimp's menus vary by location so their gluten free selections may be different than the ones below.

Appetizers

- Traditional Shrimp Cocktail

Salads

- Tossed Chicken Cobb Salad
- Pear & Berry Salad

Forrest's Favorites

- Accidental Fish & Shrimp
- Shrimp & Veggie Skewers
- Mahi Mahi & Veggie Skillet
- Steamed Broccoli
- Fresh Fish Selections (Varies by Location)
- Fresh Fish with Mango Pineapple Salsa
- Fresh Fish with Lobster Butter Sauce
- Fresh Fish Cajun Style

Kids

- Kids Grilled Chicken

Dessert

- Jenny's Mini's

Captain D'S

Entrees

- Wild Alaskan Salmon
- Wild Alaskan Salmon Salad
- Shrimp Skewers
- Premium Shrimp
- Seasoned Tilapia
- Shrimp Scampi

Sides

- Broccoli
- Sliced Cheese
- Corn on the Cobb
- Green Beans
- Side Salad
- Roasted Red Potatoes
- Baked Potatoes

Sauces and Condiments

- Sweet Chili Sauce
- Tartar Sauce
- Blue Cheese Dressing
- Honey Mustard Dressing
- Ranch Dressing
- Thousand Island Dressing
- Mayo
- Cocktail Sauce

Long John Silvers

Entrées

- Grilled Pacific Salmon
- Shrimp Scampi
- Freshside Grille® Salmon Entrée
- Freshside Grille® Shrimp Scampi Entrée

Sides

- Cole Slaw
- Corn Cobbette without Butter Oil
- Corn Cobbette with Butter Oil

- Rice
- Vegetable Medley

Condiments

- Cocktail Sauce
- Tartar Sauce
- Baja Sauce
- Louisiana Hot Sauce

Desserts

- Iceflow™ Lemonade
- Iceflow™ Strawberry Lemonade

Red Lobster

Seaside Starters

- Chilled Jumbo Shrimp Cocktail

Signature Salad

- RL Cobb Salad without dressing and croutons
- Add Chicken or Salmon to your salad

Lunch and Dinner Entrées

- Bacon-Wrapped Shrimp with mashed potatoes
- Snow Crab Legs without corn and crispy red potatoes
- Created Your Own Feat: Garlic Shrimp Scampi; Steamed Snow Crab Legs; Wood-Grilled Fresh Fish
- Shrimp You Way Scampi
- Garlic Shrimp Scampi

Four Course Feast

- Wood-Grilled Fresh Tilapia: Order without broccoli
- Toady's Fresh Fish
- Blackened or Broiled
- Grilled with Lemon Garlic Butter
- Grilled and Simply Seasoned
- King Crab Legs without corn and crispy red potatoes
- Live Maine Lobster- Steamed

Kids' Menu

- Snow Crab Legs

Desserts

- Kid's Ice Cream Sundae
- Cheesecake

Sides and Add-Ons

- Petite Shrimp to Salad Add-On
- Baked Potato
- Coleslaw
- Fresh Asparagus
- Fresh Broccoli
- Fresh Fruit- Orange Wedges
- Maine Lobster Tail Add-On
- Mashed Potatoes
- Roasted Vegetable Medley
- Snow Crab Add-On
- Dressings and Add Ons
- 100% Pure Melted Butter
- Blueberry Balsamic
- Blue Cheese Dressing
- Cocktail Sauce
- French Dressing

- Honey Mustard Dressing
- Jalapeño Ranch
- Marinara Sauce
- Pico de Gallo
- Piña Colada Dipping Sauce
- Ranch Dressing
- Red Wine Vinaigrette
- Tartar Sauce
- Thousand Island Dressing

Steakhouses

"Beef, it's what's for dinner, tonight." In this section, you'll find the gluten free menus of some of the most popular chained steakhouses across the county.

Black Angus Steakhouse

Appetizers

- Fire Grilled Fresh Artichoke
- Fire Grilled Steaks
- Top-Sirloin Center Cut
- Full Flavored Rib Eye Steak
- New York Strip Center Cut
- Filet Mignon Center Cut
- Bacon Wrapped Filet Mignon
- Steak and Seafood Partners
- Filet Mignon and Large Lobster Tails
- Filet Mignon and Grilled Prawns
- Top Sirloin and Large Lobster Tails
- Top Sirloin and Grilled Prawns

From the Sea

- Grilled King Salmon
- King Salmon and Pesto Sauce
- Fire-Grilled Prawns
- Large Lobster Tails

Chicken

- Fire Grilled Chicken

Sidekicks

- Coleslaw
- Western Wild Rice
- Classic Baked Potato
- Load Baked Potato
- Green Beans with Sautéed Bacon
- Broccoli with Parmesan Cheese

Toppers

- Sautéed Sweet Portobello Mushroom
- Sautéed Onions

Kid's Menu

- Grilled Cheese
- Sliced Top Sirloin Steak
- Grilled Chicken Breast
- Sides: Broccoli with Parmesan Cheese, Rice, or Orange Wedges

Capital Grille

Appetizers

- Wagyu Carpaccio
- Prosciutto Wrapped Mozzarella without croutons
- Oysters on the half shell
- Shrimp Cocktail
- Cold Shellfish Platter

Salads

- Caesar Salad without croutons
- Garden Salad without dressing

- The Wedge Salad
- Spinach Salad

Sides

- Roasted Crimini, Portabella, Shiitake, Oyster Mushrooms
- Baked Potatoes: typically available upon request
- Fresh Asparagus with Hollandaise
- Sams Mashed Potatoes

Entrées

Any steak ordered without sauce.

- Lamb Chops without Cherry Mostarda
- Fresh Lobster
- Fresh Seared Salmon fillet ordered without citrus glaze
- Fresh Swordfish with lemon shallot relish
- Sesame Seared Tuna
- Roasted Chicken

Dessert

- Crème Brulée
- Fresh Berries with Vanilla Cream
- Sorbet
- Flourless Chocolate Espresso Cake
- Handcrafted Ice Cream ordered without the biscotti

Charlie Brown's Steakhouse

Sharable Starters

- Garlic Mussels without garlic bread

Salads and Soups

- Chicken Caesar Salad without croutons
- French Onion Soup with no bread

Chicken

- Balsamic Chicken
- Sesame Ginger Chicken with no sauce

Prime Rib

- Duchess Cut, Queen Cut
- Charlie Cut, Double Cut

Classic Steaks

Un-topped and without frizzled onions.

- Center Cut Top Sirloin (8 oz. and 10 oz.)
- Hand-cut Filet Mignon
- Porterhouse (without onion rings)
- NY Strip (8 oz. and 12 oz.)
- 14 oz Grilled Ribeye
- Chopped Steak (no sauce)

Seafood

- Mediterranean Salmon
- Tilapia
- Cioppino (no garlic bread)
- Classic Salmon
- Grilled Salmon & Shrimp

Specialties

- Classic Cheeseburger with no bun
- Barbecue Ribs

Sides

- Fresh Steamed Asparagus
- Fresh Steamed Broccoli
- Garlic Mashed Potatoes
- Sherried Button Mushrooms
- Baked Potato
- Coleslaw
- Sauteed Onions
- Seasoned Rice
- Salad Bar Items
- All veggies
- All Salad Dressings except Asian and Ranch
- Chopped Chicken Liver
- Mozzarella & Tomato Salad
- Cottage Cheese
- Giardiniera
- Potato Salad

Sauces and Condiments

- Au Jus
- Barbecue Sauce
- Cocktail Sauce
- Creamy Parmesan Sauce
- Guacamole
- Honey Mustard
- Horseradish Sauce
- Marinara Sauce
- Melted Butter
- Orange Horseradish
- Salsa
- Sour Cream
- Steak Sauce

Fleming's Prime Steakhouse and Wine Bar

Appetizers

- Lobster Bisque Soup
- Lump Crab Louis Wraps
- Tenderloin Carpaccio: Order without croutons
- Wicked Cajun Barbecue Shrimp: Order without croutons
- Shrimp Cocktail
- Seared Ahi Tuna: Request caper creole mustard sauce

Salads

Order without croutons. All dressings are gluten free except red onion balsamic vinaigrette.

- The Wedge
- Fresh Mozzarella & Sweet Tomato
- Classic Caesar
- Fleming's Salad

Sides

- Baked Potato (all toppings are gluten free)
- Fleming's Potatoes
- Mashed Potatoes (all flavors are gluten free)
- Sautéed Spinach
- Sautéed Mushrooms
- Sautéed Sweet Corn
- Grilled Asparagus
- Roasted Baby Carrots
- Sautéed French Green Beans

Steaks

- Main Filet Mignon
- Petite Filet Mignon

- Lite Filet Mignon
- Prime Rib eye
- Prime Bone-In Rib eye
- Prime New York Strip
- Porcini Rubbed Filet Mignon
- Peppercorn Steak

Chops and Meat

- Nagle Veal Chop
- New Zealand Lamb Chops
- Double Thick Pork Rib Chop
- Double Breast of Chicken
- Prime Rib: order without au juis

Gluten Free Sauces

- Peppercorn
- Madeira
- Béarnaise
- Lemon Butter
- Lobster Sauce
- Jalapeño Pepper Sauce
- Horseradish Cream
- Horseradish Mustard
- "F17" Steak Sauce
- Champagne Mint
- Porcini Mushroom Sauce
- Smoke Jalapeño Aioli

Seafood

- Tuna Mignon
- Salmon Nicoise Salad: Order without crostini
- Seared Scallops: Order without puff pastry
- North Atlantic Lobster Tail
- Alaska King Crab Legs

Dessert

- Crème Brulée
- Mixed Berries
- Vanilla Ice Cream

The Keg Steakhouse

Starters, Salads, and Snacks

- Shrimp Cocktail
- Scallops and Bacon
- Santa Fe Chicken Dip
- Spinach Salad without pecans
- Mixed Greens Salad
- Wedge Salad with ranch dressing
- Loaded Nachos
- Surf and Turf
- Steak and Fries

Entrees

All sides are gluten free except for the rice pilaf.

- Top Sirloin Classic
- Filet Classic
- New York Classic
- Prime Rib Classic
- Grilled Top Sirloin
- Sirloin Oscar
- New York
- Baseball Top Sirloin
- Rib Steak
- Filet Mignon
- Prime Rib without frizzled onions

- Prime Rib and Tiger Shrimp
- Prime Rib and King Crab
- Prime Rib and Lobster
- Top Sirloin and Tiger Shrimp
- Top Sirloin and King Crab
- Top Sirloin and Lobster
- Zesty Salmon
- Tiger Shrimp
- Mustard Salmon
- King Crab Dinner
- Lobster Tail Dinner
- Gilled Thai Chicken
- Chicken Oscar
- Honey BBQ Chicken and Ribs
- Honey BBQ Ribs

Dessert

- Crème Brulée
- Mini Passion Fruit Brulee

LongHorn Steakhouse

Salads

Request no croutons and that the salads be tossed in separate mixing bowls from other salads.

- 7-Pepper Salad
- Chicken Caesar Salad
- Grilled Salmon Salad: Order without salmon marinade
- Mixed Green Side Salad
- Caesar Side Salad

Dressings

- House
- Ranch
- Light Ranch
- Raspberry Vinaigrette
- Balsamic Vinaigrette
- Thousand Island
- Chipotle Ranch
- Bleu Cheese
- Caesar
- Honey Mustard
- Oil and Vinegar

Burgers and Sandwiches

Must be ordered without bun

- Cheeseburger
- Bacon Cheeseburger
- Shaved Prime Rib Sandwich

Ribs, Chops, Etc.

- Babyback Ribs without BBQ sauce
- Cowboy Pork Chop

Chicken

- Sierra Chicken

Legendary Steaks

- Flo's Filet
- Bacon Wrapped Filet
- NY Strip
- LongHorn Porterhouse
- Porterhouse for Two without LongHorn Steak Sauce

- Prime Rib
- Ribeye
- Renegade Sirloin
- Fire Grilled T-Bone
- Chop Steak without red wine sauce, or crisp onion straws
- Flat Iron Steak
- Rancher's Sirloin without Bordelaise Sauce

Seafood and Steak & Seafood Combinations

All salmon must be ordered without Salmon Marinade. Order all seafood dishes without rice

- Flo's Filet and Salmon
- LongHorn Salmon
- Redrock Grilled Shrimp
- Sirloin & Redrock Grilled Shrimp
- Flo's Filet and Lobster Tail
- Grilled Fresh Rainbow Trout

Kids' Meals

- Kid's Hot Dog without bun
- Kid's Cheeseburger without bun
- Kid's Grilled Chicken salad without croutons
- Kid's Sirloin Steak
- Kid's Grilled Chicken

Flavorful Under 500 Calories

- Flo's Filet
- LongHorn Salmon
- Renegade Sirloin
- Sierra Chicken
- Grilled Fresh Rainbow Trout

Soups

- Broccoli Asiago Cheddar Soup: Order without crackers

Sides

- Baked Potato
- Mashed Potatoes
- Asparagus
- Seasonal Vegetables
- Sweet Potato
- Slice Tomatoes
- Grilled Onions
- Roasted Merlot Mushrooms: Order without sauce

Desserts

- Hot Fudge Sundae

Morton's Steakhouse

Bar Bites

- Jumbo Shrimp Cocktail
- Iceberg Wedge Bites
- Oysters on the Half Shell
- Fresh Cut Potato Chips
- Parmesan Truffle Matchstick Fries
- Blue Cheese Steak Fries

Appetizers

- Broiled Sea Scallops
- Half Dozen Oysters on the Half Shell
- Jumbo Lump Crabmeat Cocktail
- Jumbo Shrimp Cocktail

- Maine Lobster Cocktail
- Prosciutto Wrapped Mozzarella
- Chilled Ocean Platter

Soups and Salads

- Bibb Lettuce Salad
- Center Cut Iceberg with Blue Cheese Dressing
- Center Cut Iceberg with Thousand Island
- Chopped House Salad
- Chopped Spinach Salad
- Lobster Bisque
- Morton's Salad
- Sliced Beefsteak Tomato with Blue Cheese
- Sliced Beefsteak Tomato, Purple Onion Vinaigrette

Prime Steaks and Chops

- Center-Cut Filet Mignon (no au jus)
- Signature Cut Prime New York Strip (no au jus)
- Center Cut Prime Ribeye (no au jus)
- Chicago-Style Prime Bone-In Ribeye (no au jus)
- Bone-In Veal Chop
- Double-Cut Rib Lamb Chops

Upgrades

- Black Truffle Butter
- Blue Cheese Butter
- Foie Gras-Cognac Butter+

Signature Seafood

- Alaskan King Crab Legs
- Chilean Sea Bass Fillet a la Nage
- Cold Water Lobster Tail, 8 oz
- Honey-Chili Glazed Salmon Fillet

- Whole Baked Maine Lobster

Mixed Grills

- Filet Mignon
- Grilled Shrimp
- Bacon Wrapped Scallops

Side Dishes for Sharing

- Chicago Style Horseradish Mashed Potatoes
- Creamed Corn
- Grilled Jumbo Asparagus
- Hashed Brown Potatoes
- Jumbo Baked Potato, plain
- Lyonnaise Potatoes
- Parmesan & Truffle Matchstick Fries
- Sauteed Brussels Sprouts
- Sauteed Spinach & Button Mushrooms
- Sour Cream Mashed Potatoes
- Steamed Fresh Broccoli
- Steamed Jumbo Asparagus

Desserts

- Chocolate Ice Cream
- Creme Brulee
- Double Chocolate Mousse
- Fresh Raspberries
- Mixed Berries
- Raspberry Sorbet
- Vanilla Ice Cream

Outback Steakhouse

Aussie-Tizers aka Appetizers

- Seared Ahi Tuna
- Grilled Shrimp on the Barbie

Salads

- Aussie Chicken Cobb Salad: Ask for no croutons and avoid the Crispy Chicken
- California Chicken Salad
- Steakhouse Salad: Avoid the Aussie Crunch
- Chicken or Shrimp Caesar Salad: Request no croutons

Outback Favorites

Don't get Aussie Fries. Consider substituting with vegetables without seasoning or with a baked potato.

- Baby Back Ribs
- New Zealand Rack of Lamb: Avoid the Cabernet sauce
- Grilled Pork Chop
- Alice Springs Chicken
- Grilled Chicken on the Barbie
- Sweet Glazed Pork Tenderloin: Avoid crunch crumb topping

Signature Steaks

- Outback Special
- Victoria's Filet
- New York Strip
- Ribeye
- Porterhouse
- Herb Roasted Prime Rib: Avoid au jus

- ADD ONS: Grilled Scallops without Lemon Pepper Butter Sauce; Grilled Shrimp; and Lobster Tail

Perfect Combinations

Don't get Aussie Fries. Consider substituting with vegetables without seasoning or with a baked potato.

- Ribs and Chicken on the Barbie
- Filet and Grilled Shrimp on the Barbie
- Sirloin and Grilled Shrimp on the Barbie
- Filet and Lobster Tail

Straight from the Sea

- Norwegian Salmon
- Simply Grilled Mahi
- Hears of Gold Mahi: Avoid rice garnish and Lemon Pepper Butter Sauce
- Lobster Tail

Burgers and Sandwiches

Don't get Aussie Fries. Consider substituting with vegetables without seasoning or with a baked potato. Plus avoid the bread/buns.

- The Bloomin' Burger: Order without onion petals
- The Outback Burger
- Classic Cheeseburger
- Classic Cheeseburger
- Aged Cheddar Bacon Burger
- Grilled Chicken and Swiss Sandwich

Freshly Made Sides

- Fresh steamed broccoli with no seasoning
- Fresh steamed green beans with no seasoning

- Fresh seasonal mixed veggies with no seasoning
- Garlic mashed potatoes
- Dressed baked potato
- Sweet potato
- Grilled asparagus

Side Salads

Be sure to request no croutons and for the salad to be mixed in a new, separate bowl.

- Signature side salads (House or Caesar with no croutons)
- Premium Side Salads
- Classic Blue Cheese Wedge Salad: Avoid Blue Cheese Dressing
- Blue Cheese Pecan Chopped Salad: Avoid Aussie Crunch

All salad dressings are gluten free EXCEPT:

- Mustard Vinaigrette
- Blue Cheese dressing

Joey Menu aka Kid's Menu

Aussie Fries are not gluten-free

- Boomerang Cheeseburger without bun
- Joey Sirloin
- Grilled Chicken on the Barbie
- Junior Ribs
- Spotted Dog Sundae: Avoid OREO cookie crumble

Outback Specialty Cocktails

- Rita Trio
- Naturally Skinny Rita

- Suaza Gold Coast Rita
- Top Shelf Patron Margarita
- New South Wales Sangria
- The Wallaby Darned
- Sydney's Cosmo Martini

Irresistible Desserts

- Chocolate from Down Under
- Sydney's Sinful Sundae

Ruth's Chris Steakhouse

Appetizers and Soups

- Shrimp Cocktail & Shrimp Remoulade
- Barbecued Shrimp with no toast point
- Crabtini
- Seared Ahi-Tuna with no sauce

Salad Dressings

- Creamy Lemon Basil
- Thousand Island
- Remoulade
- House Vinaigrette & White Vinaigrette

Entrée Complements

- 6 Large Shrimp

Seafood

- Ahi-Tuna Stack with no sauce

Vegetables

- Fresh Asparagus with Hollandaise Sauce
- Sautéed Baby Spinach
- Fresh Broccoli
- Sautéed Mushrooms
- Broiled Tomatoes

Salads

Request that your salad is mixed in a separate bowl from all other salads

- Steakhouse Salad with no garlic croutons
- Ruth's Chop Salad with no garlic croutons & crispy onions
- Caesar Salad with no garlic croutons
- Lettuce Wedge
- Sliced Tomato and Onion

Signature Steaks and Chops

- All Steaks & Chops on our Dinner Menu are Gluten Free. Plus be sure to substitute Veal Butter from the Lamb and Veal Chops with Steak Butter

Potatoes

- Garlic Mashed
- Baked

Dessert

- Fresh Berries and Cream
- Chocolate Sin Cake
- Crème Brulee
- Ice Cream
- Sorbet

Thank You.

I'll just like to take this time and thank you so much for reading this book. I truly do hope that I was able to help make eating out on a gluten free diet at least 1% easier for you.

Thank you again for reading this book.

You rock!

P.S. *Please be sure to come say hi to me on Twitter. My username is @UrbanTastebuds*

My Websites

www.UrbanTastebuds.com

www.GlutenFreeGuideHQ.com

www.VeganRestaurantsHub.com

Social Media

Pinterest: www.Pinterest.com/AdamBryan

Twitter: www.Twitter.com/UrbanTastebuds

Instagram: www.Instagram.com/AdamBryan

36482765R00157

Made in the USA
Lexington, KY
21 October 2014